M000169904

Wrapping My Fears In Wonder

EveryDay Prayers to Help You Find, Feel, and Be Calm, Resilient, and Healthy of Mind, Body, and Spirit

Paula Strupeck Gardner

2nd Edition of EveryDay Prayers I:
Wrapping My Fears In Wonder
Includes 7 previously unpublished prayer poems.

2nd Edition: February 2021
ISBN: 978-1-7352276-1-0 (Paperback)

This volume of prayer poems has been
loved and shared by many
family, friends, and retreat participants
over the years.

To receive YOUR free recording of one of Paula's prayer
poems set to the sounds of nature or music,

Go to:
https://worthyofwingswithpaulagardner.aweb.page/
Wrapping-Your-Fears-In-Wonder

Dedication

This book is dedicated to:

My Parents, Carl and Viola Osterman Strupeck.
At the time of the first edition's publication in 2014,
They were blessing this beautiful Earth together, in their 90's,
With their own sense of wonder and joy.
Today, Mom alone carries on their legacy of exuberance in life.
We are truly blessed.

My husband,
Who helps make it possible for me to breathe
And be me;

The lights of my life —
My sons Jack and Andrew,
Aka my gurus;

And to the cherished memory of **my niece Christie Marie**
Whose laughter will live forever in my heart.

Table of Contents

Foreword

What a tremendous gift!

For those of us seeking a moment of quiet solace... of connecting with the moment, and our Indwelling Sacred Presence—especially those of us who prefer a more pragmatic, "relatable" voice than the types of lofty piety one normally encounters in prayer books and collections of spiritual reflections—Paula Gardner's *EveryDay Prayer Book* is an enriching, refreshing and welcome gift.

Enriching because her insights challenge us to return to the moment, where our perceptions are clearer, fuller, and undistracted.

Refreshing, because this collection focuses on "wrapping our fears in wonder," which is a remarkably simple, yet powerful means of opening our hearts and spirits to transformation at the deepest levels, where our fears often block us from experiencing the fullness of life.

And welcome, because we need more calm, pragmatic and centered voices to encourage us to return to the moment—the only place where we can harness the limitless potential of our personal power—and immerse our consciousness in gratitude, forgiveness, and simple presence.

The rich language of Ms. Gardner's spirituality finds clear expression in these pages, and I think in a most refreshing manner, can help to remove some of the barriers others may have previously encountered in their approaches to a more formal and less spontaneous prayer life.

These heart-felt prayers offer thanksgiving for the Beloved's caring protection, interspersed with reflections of sincere confession and longing for healing renewal, and genuine gratitude for the indwelling grace which crowns the day at sunrise, and kisses the sacred earth at nightfall.

I have had the privilege of previewing this beautiful collection personally, and am confident that it will prove to be as much of a blessing for you, as it has been for me.

Mahatma Gandhi once observed, "Prayer is not asking. It is a longing of the soul. It is daily admission of one's weakness. It is better in prayer to have a heart without words than words without a heart."

Ms. Gardner's soulful longing and humility is encouraging and inspiring, and the vulnerability with which she bares her raw pleas with the Indwelling Presence has been an invigorating experience for me and for a few folks with whom I have shared a few of her prayers.

Another gift of this collection is the fullness of joyful awareness that Ms. Gardner brings to these prayers and reflections. In his book, The Prophet, the beloved Khalil Gibran reminds us, "You pray in your distress and in your need; would that you might pray also in the fullness of your joy and in your days of abundance."

This book has been a powerful reminder, and soft-spoken, yet powerful witness, and an inspiration.

May your mornings be blessed and inspired by Ms. Gardner's gratitude. May your days be filled with simple awareness and mindfulness. And may your nights be blessed with peaceful awe and healing.

Namasté,

Khenpo Gurudas Śunyatananda, O.C., M.Sc., Th.D., N.D.
Abbot-The Contemplative Order of Compassion (Zenkondo)

Author of *Sunyata: the Transformative Power of Emptiness, Awakening: Living the Dharma of Compassion,* and *Seven Pointed Mind Training.*

Introduction and Welcome!

When you begin your day with gratitude, you open your heart and mind to receive all the grace and beauty that awaits you. When you take your everyday moments and apply to them your sense of gratitude and wonder in the form of prayer of any nature, you become your prayer.

Meister Eckhardt wrote, "If the only prayer you ever say in your life is, 'thank you,' it will be enough."

Your prayers take many forms, any forms. It can be the pause you take to watch the sun set; the smile that erupts in your heart each time you hold your baby; the softness that moves into your belly when you step onto the yoga mat away from the EveryDay and into the EveryMoment.

You're praying when you sing along with the radio as you drive and when you weep at the loss of your best friend to cancer. You're praying when you give your full attention to your partner; praying when you trip over the rug; praying when you shoot free throws and when you turn cartwheels; praying as you lie on the summer grass with your kids and find the shapes and stories in the clouds.

And you're praying when you spill your thoughts and feelings onto pages so that others may have the words to name *their* thoughts and feelings.

In this first volume of prayers, I share some of my everyday moments of fear, anxiety, anger, sadness, and confusion, and wrap them in awareness and gratitude.

The prayers appear, for the most part, in alphabetical order… just because.

I'd like to call your attention to one thing: Somewhere in the midst of writing, it dawned on me that I needed to write in a way that demonstrated taking responsibility for myself both to nurture my efforts to make that happen and to acknowledge the journey thus far. You'll know which prayers were written when because I began to use the "I" word instead of speaking in general and impersonal terms.

I invite you to place the prayers in your heart; to read the words—as they fit—with *your* voice so that you, too, can wear the mantle of "I" and own your heart's desires.

Please. Join me on this journey. Subscribe to my newsletter by going to this site:

https://worthyofwingswithpaulagardner.aweb.page/
Wrapping-Your-Fears-In-Wonder

Write to me; let me know how these prayers fit your mind/body/spirit.

All that you do, do it…with joy.

Blessings,

Paula

Prologue

"'In the beginning was the Word,' says the Gospel of St. John. What is a word? A mental image, is it not? So all that God had in the beginning was a mental image. That was His mold, and into it He poured the Creative Force all about Him and formed the world of everything upon it."

"When you pray earnestly, you form a mental image of the thing you desire and you hold it strongly in your thought. Then, if you have the necessary faith that you ARE RECEIVING the thing you asked for, your superconscious mind (which is part of the universal or God Mind), draws to you enough of the Creative Force to fill out the image you are holding in thought and to bring it into being."

From *The Secret of the Ages* by Robert Collier
©1948 Robert Collier Publications, Inc.

The Prayers

Help Me Pray.

Prayer has become the background music
    of my life.

When in doubt,
    I pray.

When in awe,
    I pray.

When I'm afraid,
    I pray.

When I'm certain,
    I pray.

Prayers of gratitude,
    prayers of forgiveness,
    prayers asking for forgiveness,
    prayers seeing guidance and clarity,
    resolve and comfort…

    cross my heart, mind, and lips
    at any given moment throughout my day.

When I was a girl,
    I loved the saying,
    "To sing is to pray twice."

Eknath Eswaren titled his book:
   Your Life Is Your Message.
My life has become a prayer,
      making prayer my message.

Blessed Mother, Holy Spirit,
      Lord Jesus,
      All the Angels and Saints and Holy Men, Women, and
            Children,

You bless my life with your presence.

In my thoughts—spoken and unspoken—
      you reside.

Please continue to shower my world
      with blessings..
      that I may learn,
      that I may give,
      that I may grow

      in love.

Help me continue to see and experience
      the value
      of recognizing beauty
      where others overlook.
Help me use my words
      to thank and honor
      the Creator, the Beloved Being beyond me.

Vygotsky believed that we thought BEFORE
      we had words.

And I believe what he saw
     was prayer.

When I meditate,
     I sometimes seek presence before words,
     beyond words.
     I seek stillness.

Stillness, like prayer, is rich with promise,
     potential.

Sometimes,
     I pray for stillness.

Ask for what you want.
     I ask for prayer.

Amen.
Blessings.

Accept the Things and People I Cannot Change.

I live to inspire people.
Having said that,
> I do not doubt that my ego loves the stroking that comes
> with seeing someone step into their life
> and believing that I had something to do with it.

HA!

People only change when they are ready to change.
If my voice happens to be around when they're ready,
> they'll hear my voice…
> but it has LITTLE to do with me
> and EVERYTHING to do with them.

Blessed Mother, Holy Spirit,
> Lord Jesus,
> All the Angels and Saints and Holy Men, Women, and
> > Children,

PLEASE
> help me let go of the notion that I can change anyone;
> that my words illuminate
> another's path
> and allow them to walk with greater confidence,
> greater vision,
> greater faith.

That does not mean
>that I will abandon my purpose of service,
>or of my desire to inspire
>others.

It DOES mean
>that I ask for your grace and guidance
>to accept that
>this person is willing to live with pain,
>that person is willing to live with fear,
>each person is free to sit still or move
>sometimes in a million different directions
>without understanding his/her divinity.

I can put the most beautiful mirror in front of them.
I cannot control or influence the image that they see.

When I provide support for them,
>help me see that it must be without any attachment
>to the results;
>and that I MAY be an instrument,
>but that it is THEY who are ready,
>open, doing whatever work they need to do.

And help me accept…
>when they pause or express…

…I can't even find the word it so distresses me…

>giving in, giving up…resigning
>themselves to whatever it is that they are experiencing.

For while my purpose may be to inspire,
 it is not my place to judge, to demean, to in any way
  dismiss.

When they're ready,
 they will hear and respond to someone's voice
  echoing their own.

Help me accept—and celebrate—the people and things
 I cannot change.

Amen.
Blessings.

Bask in the Light.

With so many challenges fighting for position in my mind,
    how about if I stop.
Look.
Listen.

Yesterday, my elder son came home from college
    for two nights and a day
    so that he could see his younger brother perform
    as one of the leads
    in a community theatre production.

Ah. Something to savor.

Late yesterday night
    (early this morning),
    they sat side by side,
    laughing at a video,
    exchanging in brotherly code.

Oh, my heart soars.

Skip over these moments?
Stay mired in worries?

Blessed Mother, Holy Spirit,
>   Lord Jesus,
>   All the Angels and Saints, and Holy Men, Women, and
>   Children,

Help me allow the warmth from the moment
>   seep into my brain, my body, and my soul.

Help me surrender to this instance of love.

Help me let go of all the other thoughts clamoring
>   for my attention.

Help me release them
>   and open my heart to the abundance
>   of loving energy emanating from the lights of my life

>   so that I might bask in this light of love
>   that each of these moments exudes.

Blessings they are.

Amen.
Blessings.

Be Glad.

Henry Van Dyke wrote,
  "Be glad of life
  because it gives you a chance
  to love, to work, to play, and to look up at the stars."

What are you glad about?
When was the last time you looked up at the stars?
When was the last time you paused to feel glad for your
    life—
    for the fact that you're breathing, for your functioning
            organs,
    including your heart and your brain and your kidneys?
When was the last time you paused
    to feel glad for your life—
    ALL of your life—
            including your family,
            your friends,
            the people you've met,
            the people who have loved you,
            the people who have hurt you,
            the mistakes you've made,
            the successes you've enjoyed?
            the pleasure you've given,
            the pleasure you've received?

When was the last time you paused
 to feel glad for your life,
 for the jobs you've had,
 the work you've done,
 the people you've helped,
 those who have helped you?

All too often,
 even in a world where we're encouraged to feel grateful,
 we save our "gratefuls" for a moment at the end of the
   day
 or at the beginning of the day
Both of those are good things to do.

I'm asking for help right now in remembering to pause
 throughout my day to be glad of life...

Blessed Mother, Holy Spirit,
 Lord Jesus,
 All the Angels, and Saints and Holy Men, Women, and
   Children,

I ask you to help me pause,
 to stop for a moment here and there
 throughout my day
 to look around
 to look within,

 and to see something for which I'm glad
 and to STOP in that gladness to breathe it in,
 to feel the smile it brings to my eyes, to my lips,
   to my heart.

I'm asking
    so that I remember
    to do more than glance at the stars in the sky.
I'm asking so that I stop and breathe in the stars in the sky,
    giving myself an opportunity
    to savor their beauty
    and the knowledge that they are part of me and I of
            them.

I'm asking
    so that I remember
    to be present when I'm playing with my kids,
    to let go of everything else on my agenda
    for that moment
    and allow myself to feel glad of life.

I'm asking
    so that I remember to
    place a loving thought in my head
    before I speak, or listen,
    or cook, or hug, or write, or read,
    or walk, or clean out the basement,
    or pick up the dishes that someone left on the table.

I'm asking
    so that gladness informs my life
    more than newspaper stories
    or memories of hurt feelings or frustration.

I'm asking
    so that I fill my life with love,
    giving love,
    receiving love,

creating love,
stirring love,
sharing love,
inspiring love…

I'm asking
so that I may remember to be glad of life,
all of life,
and to share that gladness
with all.

Amen.
Blessings.

Begin Again.

Blessed Mother, Holy Spirit, Lord Jesus,
    All the Angels and Saints, Holy Men, Women, and
        Children,

Inspire me, please, to find
    inside me
    the light that loves
    no matter what.

Guide my thoughts
    to kindness and compassion
    instead of to well-worn paths
    of impatience and intolerance.

Shine your light
    into the corners of
    my soul
    and let me see
    how my fears
    and my experiences
    are manifesting today.

Help me sweep away
    their debris,
    step over and around their dust
    and open the windows
    to let them go;

open the wounds
to let them heal.

Help me stand still and tall
as the winter winds whip
the aftermath away,

clearing me out.

to begin again.

Amen.
Blessings.

Begin with Beauty

I don't dare
    start my day
    letting my mind have its way.

I don't dare
    because it will carry me places
    I don't want to go,
    I strive not to go.

I don't dare
    because it will create a day
    filled with fear,
    sadness, anger, hostility,
    broken spirits,
    broken hearts.

I prefer, instead,
    to begin with beauty.

Before my feet even touch the floor,
    I train my mind toward gratitude—
    for another day,
    another chance
    to live with purpose, on purpose,
    to create with beauty,
    create with love.

Blessed Mother, Holy Spirit, Lord Jesus,
    All the Angels and Saints and Holy Men, Women, and
    Children,

    guide my habit-infested mind
    to a different light,
    a different room.

Help me take the steps
    that sweep my mind of the clutter
    of calamity and drama
    and replace it
    with beauty.

Help me begin with beauty
    so that I set the day
    on a trajectory
    of light and love
    instead of drab and darkness.

Instead of fear and loathing,
    turn my chin towards wisdom and hope.

Remind me to keep bedside
    inspiring volumes of prayer and insight
    so that I may quickly
    access others 'positive thoughts
    in order to nip in the bud
    any of the routine and habitual
    threads of negativity that crowd and cloud
    my desires for change

and my commitment to replacing
ugly and demeaning
with beautiful and empowering.

Guide my hands
to pick up those books
instead of a newspaper
to start my day.

Help me choose
to fill my mind with someone else's inspiration
until I can latch onto my own.

Help me ride the wave of lightness
into my day
so that I may share laughter with those I meet
throughout my day;
so that I may share peace
with those whose paths I cross;
so that I may inspire in them
the choice to
literally change their mind
to pathways
of positive expectations and abundance.

Mother Teresa said,
"Let no one come to you without leaving better and happier."

Let me imprint those words
and other words of loving kindness
in this brain
and, each day, let me begin with beauty....

and the rest of the day will follow.

Amen.
Blessings.

Breathe the Anxiety Away.

Do you ever wake up with your mind racing
    to a million places all at once
    and a gnawing in your stomach
    that has nothing to do with hunger and
    a tightening in your chest and throat?

It happens.

I can feel my throat constricting,
    my chest caving in,
    my whole body aching to go into a fetal position
    as my instinct is to protect myself.

YET I KNOW
    that I need to do the opposite of what seems to be
    natural and instinctive.

I need to draw on my intellect and knowledge and
    experience and faith…

    and BREATHE.

Blessed Mother, Holy Spirit,
    Lord Jesus,
    All the Angels and Saints and Holy Men, Women, and
        Children,

Please help me recognize these moments of anxiety
        and rather than succumb to them,
        rather than hide and run and cower before them,
        rather than turn into a ball of fear,

        help me sit with myself
        and pay attention to the anxiety:
        where do I feel it?
        where is it from?

Acknowledge.

And then breathe…slowly, long, evenly, and deeply.

Help me visualize my breath moving the length
        of this frightened, tensing body
        and help me allow the breath
        to soften these tightening muscles,
        these anxious limbs.
        Remind me
        that denying the anxiety and fear
        NEVER helps alleviate it;
        rather,
        it feeds the stress,
        feeds the anxiety,
        feeds the fear,
        feeds the fetal position that
        keeps threatening to take over.

Help me remember that
        bringing attention to a body part
        softens that body part
        and that each successive softening

contributes to my ability
to relax.

And refocus on this moment.

It turns my heart, my eyes, my mind
to
now
and away from what was
or what I feared was;
away from what might be
or what I fear might be.

Breathe.
It sounds so simplistic and trite,
so trendy.

But it's true
that wiser people than I have used the breath
for thousands of years
to calm anxiety,
to cool anger,
to soothe and soften stressing minds and bodies.

And it's true
that our modern science now affirms
this wisdom as real.

Help me breathe away the anxiety
when it insinuates itself into my core.
Help me breathe away the anxiety
when it rounds my shoulders
and bows my head.

Help me breathe through it,
    around it, into it…

Help me breathe myself back to today.

Amen.
Blessings.

Breathe Through The Day.

Breathe through today…

I didn't say BREEZE…
    although that idea can be very appealing…

Imagine:
    sailing through traffic, through work,
    through altercations,
    through meal prep,
    through endless waiting in line,
    through bedtimes, through story times,
    through books and papers and calls, oh my!

No.
I didn't say BREEZE.

I KNOW that when I'm in the moment
    and doing what I love
    for those I love, it doesn't feel like work.
I don't feel a need to get to BREEZE.

It IS a breeze to live life loving every moment.

What I'm asking for is help to BREATHE
    through the day.
Blessed Mother, Holy Spirit,
    Lord Jesus,

All the Angels and Saints and Holy Men, Women, and
Children,

Help me BREATHE.

Help me take
a slow, long, even, deep breath IN
and feel every moment of that intake of breath.
Help me feel each cell responding to the depth
and breadth of that breath.

Help me take a long, slow, even deep breath OUT
and feel every moment of that release of breath.
Help me feel each cell responding
to the loosening of breath as it allows the body
to let go of tension, tightness, emotions...

Help me watch, listen, feel the breath moving
in and out of the body, moving each moment,
moving ME in each moment.

Help me breathe through traffic.
Help me breathe through
contentious moments
and people in my day.

Help me breathe through
annoying but necessary tasks.

Help me breathe through
the anxiety
that keeps me from savoring each moment with each
person

near and dear to me
because I'm thinking of all the other things I must do.

Help me breathe through
    the distractions that pop up
    on-and offline as I work.

Help me breathe through
    the disappointments
    with myself and with others.

Help me breathe through
    pain that pops up or persists
    that I may listen and let go and take care of.

Help me breathe through
    unpleasant or difficult conversations
    so that I may be responsible
    and do what I must do.

Help me breathe through
    the reluctance
    that plagues me when I have to do something
    that challenges me
    for whatever reason
    but that I must do if I'm to learn or move forward
    or succeed.

Help me breathe
    through someone else's words
    so that I may LISTEN with greater
    attention and fuller awareness.

Help me breathe
    my impatience with myself and others
    and processes and trip-ups and bureaucracies
    and…and…and…

Help me breathe through
    life
    so that I may LIVE life.

Amen.
Blessings.

Carve out time.

There was a period of time...
    when I gave myself 30 minutes every morning to sit
        quietly
    to breathe and be,
    to "meditate."

There was a time...
    when I gave myself 15 minutes every morning to sit
        quietly
    to breathe and be,
    to set my intentions for the day.

I have meditated
    off and on for 35 years or so.
I have enjoyed years at a time
    when I carved out a portion of my day
    every day
    to practice yoga and meditation.

Sometimes,
    I sat for 5 minutes,
    sometimes, 35.
Sometimes, my yoga practice
    was active,
    sometimes restorative.

But it was a gift to myself
    that helped me give to those I love.

I felt
    centered,
    better able to listen without reacting,
    without judging,
    without otherwise making a fool of myself.

I'm not sure when I lost that discipline,
    focus,
    self-care.

I need to cultivate again
    whatever it was that allowed me to
    carve out a space in the day for me
    to be quiet;
    to empty myself of thoughts
    (This is no easy feat, is it?)

Blessed Mother, Holy Spirit,
    Lord Jesus,
    All the Angels and Saints and Holy Men, Women, and
        Children,

I need your help.

What I remember as seeming natural,
    now seems forced.

And I need your blessings and your nudge
    to help me find that path again
    or create a new one.

Please help me make, schedule,
>   write on the calendar
>   at least 15 minutes every day
>   that is mine to sit and breathe and be.

Soothe my fears
>   that I'll not get everything done.
Remind me
>   that this quiet time
>   allows me to be more efficient,
>   more focused,
>   better able to do what I need to do
>   without distraction.

Nudge me, please,
>   to recall that when I give myself this time,
>   I am so much better able to
>   give to others what they need
>   rather than react to what they say
>   or don't say;
>   help me recognize anew
>   that this time inside
>   eases my ability
>   to respond instead of react;
>   to let go of what isn't mine;
>   to accept responsibility for what is.

Lead me
>   to remember the words of Thich Nhat Han who wrote:

>   *"We are here to take care of each other;*
>   *to do so, we must first take care of ourself."*

and to set aside this time
of drawing my attention
again and again and again and again—
however many times it takes—
to stillness.

Help me step away
and step in.

Help me see
and breathe
and be.

Amen.
Blessings.

Clarity.

Blessed Mother, Holy Spirit,
    Lord Jesus,
    All the Angels and Saints and Holy Men, Women, and
        Children,

Help me live in the light of awareness.

As I begin this day,
    help me identify, help me discern
    what it is that I long for,
    what it is that I seek.

Help me quiet the doubts that
    prevent me from seeing clearly
    the desires that drive me.

Help me brush aside the
    veils of fear that distort what I do see.

Help me look in the right places,
    perceive what's really there
    and receive the vision as mine.

Help me shine a light on all I see;
    to cut through the distortions

    and head straight into my heart of hearts

to identify what's there

and then, to live what's there with love.

Amen.
Blessings.

Compassion for Others.

Blessed Mother, Holy Spirit,
    Lord Jesus,
    All the Angels and Saints and Holy Men, Women, and
        Children,

I pray today for compassion.

Help me see beyond me.
And hear the pain or frustration or fear
    in others' voices;
    help me see it in their eyes;
    or in the furrow of their brow;
    or in their stillness.

Help me feel this compassion in my heart of hearts.

I know that when I'm present with them
    in this moment,
    and not thinking about all that I have to do
    or where I need to go;

When I'm present with them,
I'm not judging or criticizing.

So, help me be present with them in their struggle
    no matter how
    it breaks my heart to see them like this.

It isn't about me.

Help me be ok with an awareness of how I'm feeling,
    but focused on how it's their pain,
    their fear,
    their frustration,
    their struggle.

And at this moment,
    help me remember
    that I'm here to be here
    for them.

Help me put compassion
    in the forefront of my mind;
    help me set that intention
    so that I may speak and listen and touch
    from a place of genuine compassion
Without considering its benefit to me.

Help me be here

For them.

Amen.
Blessings.

Confidence.

Blessed Mother, Holy Spirit,
    Lord Jesus,
    All the Angels and Saints and Holy Men, Women, and
        Children,

Please. Grant me the confidence
    that comes from
    deep down inside;

    confidence that is born not of arrogance,
    but of quiet personal awareness;

    confidence in one's self, one's motives,
    one's intentions;

    confidence that comes from knowledge
    of one's strengths and skills,
    as well as one's needs and wants,
    sometimes called shortcomings,
    as though there were a perfect model to fall short of.

Let me not waver
    as some around me push those buttons
    that challenge confidence,
    calling it all into question,
    as though my awareness

were inadequate, incomplete,
incorrect.

Inspire me to use this confidence
to help others gain theirs.

Even when they do not trust my intentions,
let me believe in them, in me,
knowing that my intentions
are part of my heart.

Amen.
Blessings.

Create Energy.

Blessed Mother, Holy Spirit,
    Lord Jesus,
    All the Angels and Saints and Holy Men, Women, and
        Children,

I come to you today to ask for help
    as I work to create and sustain energy
    to live and love,
    to be present for those I love
    or at least like
    and even for those whose paths I cross
    without exchanging affection.

Help me recognize and act
    on those things that I know
    (but don't always do)
    will help me create and sustain energy
    throughout my day.

Help me choose my food
    with attention and care,
    selecting as often as I'm able
    organic, real food
    that will help me be healthy.
Help me eat well throughout the day
    and to sit down while I eat,
    pausing in my day

to express gratitude to those who grew the food,
those who processed, sold, and prepared it.

Help me enjoy my treats
without having to enjoy the whole batch.

Help me exercise daily—
a short walk goes a long way
in helping me think clearly and creatively,
breathe deeply, and generate energy
for all that I choose to do.
And don't always make time.
Help me make time.

Help me spend time outdoors—
no matter the weather—
to sustain my connection to Nature
and its healing and inspiration.

Help me breathe
deeply and evenly
especially out
to clear the lungs of stale breath
so that I can take in more new, fresh breath
to keep me going strong.

Help me take care of myself
through the little, daily rituals
of cleansing and nurturing.

Help me find joy
in all things.

Help me laugh an honest,
    pure, fun-loving laugh,
    and never at anyone else's expense.

Help me focus on what I'm doing while I'm doing it
    so that my energy stays directed
    rather than scattered and, therefore,
    undermined.

Help me soften my death grip
    on keys, books, bags, the steering wheel.
Help me release the tension from my jaw,
    my shoulders, my back, my legs, my hands,
    my forehead.
That tension saps my energy.
When I soften,
I only use the energy that I need for what I'm doing

        and then all the other things that I'm doing to build my
                energy
        are infinitely more successful.

Help me make time to sit quietly
    with those I love,
    including by myself,
    be it with a good book,
    with the piano,
    or a gentle conversation
    about the day,
    or soft, loving silence.

All these things,
>   I know help me create energy
>   that help me live and love fully.
Help me do them,
>   consistently —
>   day in and day out —
>   so that I may
>   rejoice
>   in each day that the Lord has made.

Amen.
Blessings.

Cultivate Expansiveness.

What?!
Why on earth would I want to expand any more than
    I have over the last several years?

Not that kind of expansion.

Have you ever felt so overwhelmed by fear and anxiety
    that all you wanted to do was shut down?
    gather yourself and those you love closer and closer in?
    circle the wagons to protect all that you are and have?

I believe that, for many of us,
    that IS the natural inclination when we face things
    that scare us.

Business falls off while bills keep piling up.

Yes, indeed, we need to pay attention and choose wisely —
    our thoughts as well as our words and our actions.

But the common mistake we make
    is to hold our breath,
    gather in all our cards and hold them so close to our
        chest
    that even we cannot see them.

We focus on our worry and our doubt.
We withhold.
We see only the shadows
and not the light
shining behind and within us that creates those
shadows.
We are so focused on what we don't have or want
that we attract more of that to us.
We lose sight of all that we're grateful for
and we put our attention on what we're afraid of.

And we, therefore, draw more of that to us.

Blessed Mother, Holy Spirit,
Lord Jesus,
All the Angels and Saints and Holy Men, Women, and
Children,

Pleeeeeease help me remember the forest.
Pleeeeeease help me take deep, cleansing, renewing breaths.
Pleeeeeease help me cultivate a mindset of abundance
and remember that where I put my attention
is what I'll get more of.
Guide me as I trip over and around
my worries and anxieties.

Help me stumble past them and remember
that we create our life;
that I'm creating a life of expansiveness,
of love,
of success,
of beauty and goodness,
of wealth of all kinds.

Help me focus beyond this trying and troubling moment
    to see and embrace my vision;
Hold my hand to help me navigate this path
    strewn with doubt
    to continue moving with faith toward my belief.

Help me let go of the fretting so that I can
    act with confidence.

Help me release my fears
    of what may happen
    and embrace my vision
    of what may happen
    so that I create what I want to happen
    rather than what I fear.

Help me expand beyond these fears,
    beyond these worries.
Help me expand my mind and heart
    to where I intend to be
    and see clearly the highway that gets me there.

Help me remember what I believe
    and take the actions
    and choose the words
    that will support those events.

Help me expand my lungs with breath,
    my mind and heart with vision,
    my body with actions to make happen
    what I believe.

I see what I believe in.
I become what I believe.

Amen.
Blessings.

Dance!

So often,
>we plod through our life—
>one labored step at a time,
>leaving heavy footprints of effort and routine and
>>drudgery.

What if…?
We lightened our step
>with a lilt of laughter?
>with a heartfelt smile?
>with a song on our lips and in our heart and in our
>>voice?

What if we danced through our life?
Still one step at a time, certainly,
>but one joy-filled step,
>one melody-filled step,
>one feel-good-all-over step
>that carried us into each day?

Blessed Mother, Holy Spirit,
>Lord Jesus,
>All the Angels and Saints and Holy Men, Women, and
>>Children,

Help me lift my knees and kick up my feet
     in the joy of breathing in the morning,
     another day,
     another joy-filled day!

Take my hand
     and twirl me around each moment
     so that I may feel its joy.

Dos-y-dos
     with me as I hug all those I love
     and gather them into this dance of life,
     this life-filled dance.

Turn my head so that I may see the wonder.
Smile with me
     as I look around in awe
     at all the beauty,
     all the majesty.

Tickle me with your infectious laughter
     so that I may join in
     and love each day as it arises and arrives.
Guide my steps
     into a joyful cadence.

Help me find the beautiful
     rhythm and song
     of each moment
     so that I may dance along.

Shall we?

Amen.
Blessings.

Dedicate My Day.

I have found when I teach yoga
    that setting an intention acts as an anchor:
    we can come back to that intention
    again and again
    throughout our practice
    to center our mind/body/spirit.

So it can be also
    with each day that I'm given.

I can set an intention
    or dedicate my day
    to a specific person or goal or desire.

Blessed Mother, Holy Spirit,
    Lord Jesus,
    All the Angels and Saints and Holy Men, Women, and
        Children,

Help me remember at each day's dawning
    to think and speak out loud
    an intention for my day.

Help me dedicate my day
    to exercising more patience
    or speaking with loving kindness
    or refocusing my attention on my work

or listening without an agenda
or in thoughts of another person
who may need that attention or prayer.

Help me see and experience the value it brings
to give myself to one thought,
one task,
one person
each day.

Help me see the value in centering myself
so that I think, speak, move from that center
throughout my day.

Help me use that dedication
as my anchor, returning again and again
to that center.

I know that attention to a muscle
brings softness
and attention to an idea
brings it to its fruition.

Please help me apply what I know,
do what I intellectually am aware of.

Help me dedicate my day
to someone who needs the attention
or the prayers.
Help me dedicate my day
to something I need to do
to be my truest, highest self.

Help me dedicate my day
      to you.

Amen.
Blessings.

Embrace It All.

We tend to shy away from pain and sadness.
We don't talk about death.
We avert our eyes and our heart when we see
    or feel
    suffering.

What we really need to do
    is embrace the pain and suffering,
    the sadness that makes us want to crawl into a hole
    and hide under the covers,
    wishing the world away.

When we embrace the sadness,
    we also embrace the people who are experiencing that
        sadness.
Putting it on the table
    allows us all to see it, feel it,
    look at it.
When we can talk about it,
    even saying, "I don't know what to say,"
    we open the possibilities
    of healing,
    of growth.

When we hold the sadness in our hands,
    we can examine its hold on our hearts

and from there,
we can love our way back
to a place where joy awaits.

Blessed Mother, Holy Spirit,
    Lord Jesus,
    All the Angels and Saints and Holy Men, Women, and
        Children,

Open my eyes and my heart
    to pain and sadness.

Help me sit softly with them
    and with the people who feel them,
    including myself.

Help my ears open to the depths of their despair.
Help me speak of pain with the deepest compassion.
Help me words flow from my heart to theirs
    as they live through their moment of profound sadness.

Help me remember that, in order to know the light,
    we must experience the dark.
Help me embrace the darkest corners
    so that I may embrace the light
    that shines from them and into them.

Help me embrace it all.

Amen.
Blessings.

Forgiveness 1

How do I forgive others when I'm unable to forgive myself?
I say, "I'm sorry."
But my heart remains heavy with remorse,
     guilt, regret.

Blessed Mother, Holy Spirit,
     Lord Jesus,
     All the Angels and Saints and Holy Men, Women, and
          Children,

Help me know and accept my responsibility;
Help me also know the release
     of forgiveness—

     of letting go of the blaming and shaming that
     I relentlessly rain upon my head and heart.

How does it happen that we are so relentless
     in our self-criticism?

It happens sometimes that I blame
     even when there is no blame;

     that I perceive a wrong in myself
     where there is none.

Help me release the weight
    of that perceived wrong;

Help me ease the pain
    of imagination misguided;

And at those moments and at the times
    when I HAVE hurt someone,

Guide my steps
    to the open door where forgiveness beckons
    to the freedom
    of seeing ourselves
    with the same loving eyes
    with which we see others.

Forgive.
Learn.
Let go of all but the lesson.

Amen.
Blessings.

Forgiveness II.

Blessed Mother, Holy Spirit,
    Lord Jesus,
    All the Angels and Saints and Holy Men, Women, and
        Children,

Forgive me.
Forgive me for hurting others
    with my thoughtless words, silences, actions,
    inactions;
    my oversights and overdrafts,
    my inattention
    and my insensitive insistences.

Forgive me when I've hurt someone unknowingly.

Help me forgive myself for being imperfect,
    for being human
    so that I may one day
    not need to forgive myself
    or others
    for our human-ness.

Help me forgive myself
    for my unbelieving ways
    and for my fears that keep me
    from living the life I love.

Guide my steps
 toward
 forgiving those who have wounded me
 intentionally and unintentionally—with their sharp
  words,
 glares, unawareness
 or silence.

Help me ask others
 for their forgiveness and help me hear them out
 as they express and unburden
 so that we may
 all heal.

Help us heal.
And crawl back to the light
 of an open
 and clear heart
 emptied of all
 but love,
 making room
 for all the light and love
 that surrounds us
 and fills us

 once we empty ourselves
 of all
 that we need to forgive

 and all that needs to be
 forgiven.

Amen.
Blessings

Get DOING.

I have so many great ideas!
I have so many projects swirling around in my head.
I'm inspired by something every day.

And I'm grateful that I'm able to embrace the world
    as I do and think of ways to share that beauty with
        others…

And here's the but…

What am I DOING about these great ideas?

I've heard it said—
    and I believe—
    that we each have at least one book inside of us.

Well,
I have lots.
And some of them are already in my computer.
Many more are bubbling in my head and heart.

I really do want others to read what I write;
I really want to inspire others to share their gifts;
I really want to lead others to create the life they love.

Right?

So, what am I DOING to make that happen?

Blessed Mother, Holy Spirit,
    Lord Jesus,
    All the Angels and Saints and Holy Men, Women, and
        Children,

Kick me in the butt, please,
    to get me doing.

Whatever courage, confidence, or commitment I need,
    please stir it up inside of me.

So that I can make the call
    or write the email,
    or follow the program
    to get published, to get coaching,
    to get scheduled…

Help me run through whatever it is that is blocking my way
    or run around it, if that would work better.
Push me past
    the last few paragraphs of the book,
    the last few exercises of my studies,
    the final feet of my funrun/walk.

Pull me into motion
    so that I complete what I've created in my mind
    and heart.

Ideas are beautiful.
Making them real?
Sublime.

Help me get doing.

Amen.
Blessings.

Go All In!

Helen Keller wrote:

> *"Life is either a daring adventure*
> *or nothing at all."*

I don't get the benefits of a 30-minute swim by sticking
    my big toe in to test the water.

I don't get healthier by buying a pair of running shoes
    and leaving them in the closet.

I don't grow by looking repeatedly
    at personal development programs
    and then shrugging my shoulders and saying,
    "next time" or "later" or "not today."

Why not today?
What's wrong with now?

Blessed Mother, Holy Spirit,
    Lord Jesus,
    All the Angels and Saints and Holy Men, Women, And
        Children,

Help me slice through this resistance,
    well-meaning as it is,
    to DO what I meant do do.

Help me recognize the value
     of jumping in and getting started
     with dedication and persistence and
     commitment and determination.

Help me recognize MY value
     and realize that 'tis I
     that is worth the jumping in,
     the dedication, the commitment
     and determination.

When I start looking around,
     doubting myself, wondering if I'm being foolish,
     turn my eyes back to the prize—me—
     so that I may tune out
     all the critics, the would-be experts,
     those who have been like me,
     meaning to do something,
     but always choosing something or someone else
     first.

Help me choose me this time.
Lead me right into the fray,
     right into the fire
     because that's where the phoenix flies from.

Take me right into the belly of this beast
     that I call fear
     and that masquerades as "being realistic"
     or "sensible."

What greatness was ever accomplished
     by being sensible?

Help me trust my gut.
Help me see beyond where I am
 to where I will soar
 when I jump in—feet or head first doesn't matter,
 even a belly-flop will do—
 to working on myself,
 working on my projects,
 working on my dreams.

Please help me lift these weights
 off my shoulders, off my heart,
 and
 feel how the fires of passion
 drive me higher, wider, faster, farther, deeper...

Go all in.

Or not at all.

As Yoda said, "Do or do not. There is no trying."

Go all in. Give me a push, please.

> *"Come to the edge, he said.*
> *We are afraid, they said.*
> *Come to the edge, he said.*
> *They came to the edge,*
> *He pushed them and they flew."*
>
> —Apollinaire

Amen.
Blessings.

Grant Me The Serenity.

...to accept the things (and people) I cannot change;
the courage to change the things (can't change people) I
can; and the wisdom to know the difference.

(Adapted from The Serenity Prayer)

Torn between speaking up,
    tearing my hair and heart out,
    and exercising patience and equanimity..or the desire
        thereof,
I sit. And stand. And walk.
Back and forth across the floor,
across the week.

Life changes.
We age. We grow old.
Very old if we're lucky enough.

And life and age
    bring changes to our mind/body/spirit.

Are you ready?
Doesn't matter.

The changes come.
Can you manage it?
Of course, you can.

You've managed everything in your life so far.

Still, the sensation that you want
     to make it better nags at you as you listen or watch or
          both;
     you want to jump in and do for others what they
     either need to learn to do for themselves
     or can no longer do for themselves…as well
     (or as quickly) as you'd like.

Some people may not experience this conflict,
     but I do.

And so I ask:
Blessed Mother, Holy Spirit,
Lord Jesus,
     All the Angels and Saints and Holy Men, Women, and
          Children,

Please guide my words and actions
     to a place of watchful and ready attention;
     please help me support, without doing;
     enthuse, without patronizing;
     acknowledge, without judging or shaming or criticizing.
Dynamite is weak
     compared to the dynamics of family and friends
     when it comes to change,
     when it comes to letting go;
     when it comes to…living and letting live.

I pray for the serenity to live and let others live;
    to know when to step in and on toes
    (Is it inevitable?)
    and when to come around through the back door.

Peace, I wish for you.
My peace I give to you.

Let it be mine.
Let it be yours.
Let it be theirs.

Amen.
Blessings.

It All Counts.

I'm coming up to an anniversary of sorts.
A year ago this week,
    I took the decision to step out
    of my comfort zone
    and pursue myself from a totally different
    perspective
    than I had to that date.

It was a great experiment.

And I have grown.

Life changes our views
    when we change our life,
    whether we experience that change
    as a dramatic departure from
    who we've been
    or as a minuscule moment of insight.
It all counts
    because each contributes
    to where we are right now.

While we're in the throes of the decision
    that leads to the step we take,
    it can feel as though the world's waves
    are crashing around, on, over, and in us.

And then we step into the water
    and it feels...good or right or...not.

We only know when we take that step.
And the guarantee is
    that there is no guarantee.

Before I try on a coat,
    I choose the color I like,
    I choose the style I like
    from looking at it from the outside.

Until I slip my arms into the sleeves
    and feel the weight across my upper back
    and look in the mirror,
    I cannot know
    how it will feel, how it will look to my eyes,
    how it will fit, how I will like it from the inside.

And truth be told,
    I may be able to wear it for several seasons
    and then not—
    because I change
    either my tastes or my body or I wear it out.

As I look back over the year,
    I smile at how that step has changed me
    and then I smile because
    that step was connected
    to all that came before
    in some way or another.

It all matters.
It's the things behind the one thing
  that propel us into THE STEP.

I long—as I always do—
  to hold onto the experience
  and the people;
  to hold the sun, the inspiration,
  the excitement, the gratification,
  the gratitude in my hands and in my heart
  forever!

But that coat no longer fits
  and it's time for me to let it go,
  to sigh at its former loveliness
  and at my excitement in its then uniqueness.

So, I ask for help
  in emptying the pockets,
  tenderly releasing thoughts and words
  and people to their own places,
  gently soothing disappointments,
  shoring up the inner strengths
and resolves that surfaced,
holding to my heart
the hearts that continue to harmonize
with my soul's song.

Blessed Mother, Holy Spirit,
  Lord Jesus,
  All the Angels and Saints and Holy Men, Women, and
    Children,

help me hang this painting
on the wall of my mind
reserved for life-affirming landscapes.

Help me recognize its singular beauty
and realize the dreams that led me to that moment.

Help me embrace
in its totality
the scrambled path that wound its way
through life to that moment of shaking off
fear
so that I could step into
an expanded version
of me.

It was a different road than I expected.

It led me to friendships and information
and unparalleled transformations
that would not have happened
in quite the same way
without that step.

Help me appreciate all of that—
without bitterness or self-doubt;
with a warm, quiet gaze and a soft smile.

Help me see
or at least appreciate
the greater plan, the larger view,
the unfolding nature of my life

and how I choose the steps
if not the path.

Help me embrace what was,
   what is, and what will be
   in this beautiful tapestry of life.

Ah…a coat of many colors is my life.
Each, an integral partner of the other.

Help me always be open
   to tasting what can be tasted,
   seeing what can be seen

   with gratitude for all and every.

Amen.
Blessings.

It's Up To Me.

We live in a world where many of us feel entitled.
We look around and we see others doing
    what we want to be doing,
    having what we want to have,
    wearing what we want to wear,
    driving what we want to drive,
    going where we want to go…

We see what we don't have.
We rue what we have or did
    or how our parents or brothers or sisters
    or teachers or coaches or playmates or classmates
    or teammates or friends
    neglected us, berated us, shamed us,
    ignored us, betrayed us, denied us,
    ridiculed us, hurt us…

The past is passed.

What happens today
    is. up. to. me.

Blessed Mother, Holy Spirit,
    Lord Jesus,
    All the Angels and Saints and Holy Men, Women, and
        Children,
I beseech thee:

Help me take responsibility for me.
Wholehearted. Full. No excuses.
Responsibility for who I am, what I do, what I choose,
    who I'm with
    today.

Help me stand up
    and claim my life as mine.
Help me see, accept, and rejoice
    that if it's to be, it's up to me.

Tell me to look beyond my frowns and furrows,
    beyond my tears and pouty lips;
    to listen beyond my whines and moans,
    beyond my grudges and sobs.

Show me how I can make the sun shine
    in my heart
    on the cloudiest and grayest of days;
    how I can step up and step out
    of where I came from
    and run to where I want to be.

Help me close my ears
    to the cries and whispers and shouts
    that tried to drown out my dreams
    and help me reclaim them
    or create new ones
    even BIGGER and WIDER and MORE GLORIOUS
    than my originals.

Help me heal from the wounds
    that the silence knifed into me.

Help me walk tall and proud and full of purpose.
Smile on me
    as I smile at the world around me,
    confident that what I make of it
    is up to me.

Help me neither deny nor blame
    my roots for how they made my flowers falter.
But help me make of them
    a new garden,
    a vibrant, lush garden
    of love and life and time.

Mine. Help me make it mine.
Help me create the life I love.

Help my eyes see clearly,
    yesterday's veils swept away,
    as I step gingerly, then walk,
    then run,
    arms spread wide, the bliss inside
    welcoming the bliss outside.

Help me let go of the scars, the hurts,
    the angers, the pain.

Help me see:
It's up to me.
Words from my mind, my heart, my lips.
It's up to me.

Amen.
Blessings.

Leaving it to God

Over the weekend,
    my son visited from college.
When we brought him back there—
    to what he now calls home—
    we had a bit of a tiff
    over whether or not he needed help
    carrying things.

He did not need our help.
We needed to help him.

It reminded me of his two-year-old self
    proclaiming that he could do it himself.
It reminded me of how
    I only learned to accept help
    when I was as a big as a house,
    pregnant with one,
    carrying another.

I learned that it was better than ok
    to accept help.
    It was good.

Good for me.
Good for the person offering.

I learned to pause
    and allow others to enjoy
    the gift of helping me;
    whether or not I needed help
    was immaterial.

And as I write these words,
    it dawns on me.

And I ask for help.

Blessed Mother, Holy Spirit, Lord Jesus,
    All the Angels and Saints and Holy Men, Women, and
            Children,
    help me let God and His Universe
    take care of these things
    over which I have no control.

Guide me
    as I let my son figure out his own life.

Help me understand that he, like me,
    has to trip over his own feet
    in order to stand on them.

And help me, once I understand,
    to act on that understanding
    and let him make his own mistakes.

Help me not cringe too loudly
    when he stumbles,
    and embrace the stumbles as gifts
    of learning.

And help me see past me,
    around my eyes,
    to him.

Help me celebrate his triumphs
    not as mine
    but as his.

For he is not mine.

He belongs to the Universe.

What he accomplishes
    may reflect me in some way
    but it is all his.

It is up to him
    to learn, as Isaac Newton said,
    to honor the giants
    on whose shoulders he stands
    that allow him to see beyond
    what was seen before.

Help me embrace
    that, while wobbly, he is, indeed,
    standing on his own two feet,
    creating the life he loves.

And help me
    as I wobble
    in learning to stand even more to the side
    of his side,
    arms pinned to my side,

ıg God and His Universe
y my love's energy
ı heart
ᵤₐₜ ne may use it
as needed.

Or not.

Amen.
Blessings.

Let It Come.

Each moment of each day is unique
    and asks of us a unique response.

Am I prepared to respond to each unique moment?

Or am I plodding along the path,
    acting out of habit?

Good habits are good things.
We NEED to learn, develop, integrate
    good habits into our lives
    so that we can act on good habits
    instead of bad.

Bad habits?
I'll bet you have ONE!

Procrastinating.
Avoiding exercise.
Keeping silent when I see something wrong.
Demeaning myself.
Speaking in negative ways.
Using words that depress or shame instead of inspire.
Doing everything but what I intend to do.
(You know, for example, that if I'm cleaning the house
it's because I had wanted to do something productive
that I'm procrastinating about.)

Picking up the phone while I'm driving (Boy! did that
    become a habit quickly!)
Choosing chocolate over an apple.
(Is that really a bad habit?)
Making fun of myself.
Waiting to take the dog for a walk until...?
Saving my yoga practice for later in the day.
Delaying a phone call that needs to be made.

Hmmm. That's interesting.
Many seem to stem from procrastinating.
Putting off taking care of myself.,
    delaying what I love to do, want to do,
    know is good for me and for others.

So, one might think that I was praying for a nudge to DO!
But I'm praying to learn how to let it COME to me.

Blessed Mother, Holy Spirit,
Lord Jesus,
    All the Angels and Saints and Holy Men, Women, and
        Children,

Help me sit with my anxiety
    and let some of life come to me.

Help me see that running after things, people, ideas,
    projects, etc.
    is not always appropriate in this moment.

Help me believe that the best action for a given moment
    is...inaction.

Balance is a prayer for another day.
So is knowing when to act and when not to act.

THIS prayer is this: Let It Come To Me.

Let the answers come.
Let the meditation come.
Let the love come.

I spend a lot of my day chasing…
    chasing kids, chasing appointments, chasing errands,
    chasing work, chasing words,
    chasing ideas,
    chasing…

What if…

What if I sit quietly in this moment
    and let the moment come to me?
    let the words come to me?
    let others have the opportunity to know the satisfaction
    of doing?

Help me see and trust the value
    in giving myself time each day to
    let it come to me…

Whatever it is…
Let it come.

Amen.
Blessings.

Let It Come To Me.

"Strive to make all life better and you will have all Life's power backing you."

—Victor Wooten in *The Music Lesson*.

"Do more than you get paid for and eventually, you'll get paid for more than what you do."

—Unknown.

I am a very impatient woman.
I like to make things happen.

This is all good.
Except when it isn't.

Some things and people
    need to be allowed to come to me.

Making things happen
    needs to be balanced with listening
    and watching
    and letting happen.

As a parent,
    I watch my sons
    and I am learning, learning, learning
    to watch and wait and listen

They must create their own lives now.
It's no longer my job to make things happen.
It's theirs.

Where do I step in and when do I wait?
Or not?

Lao Tsu wrote:

> *"Do I have the patience to wait
> until the mud settles and the water is clear;
> to remain unmoving until the right action
> occurs on its own?"*

Well, my instantaneous answer is a resounding, "NO!"

But that doesn't mean I don't want to learn how to listen,
    how to discern, how to balance;
    how to let it come to me.

I do.

That doesn't mean that I believe I must sit,
    do nothing

(although that, too, can be sometimes true)
    and expect the world to come to me.

Blessed Mother, Holy Spirit,
Lord Jesus,
    All the Angels and Saints and Holy Men, Women, and
        Children,

Help me take a deepening breath
    and recognize the possibility
    that when I set a goal,
    I must then focus on doing the work
    and not on the end result.

Instead of obsessing about the end,
I need to write down what I need to do
    and then not wait but allow the results to happen,
    to stay out of the way so that what I worked on
    can occur.

Help me recognize
    that I must honor others' lives
    as theirs;
    that when someone asks for advice,
    what they often desire is someone to hear them,
    to listen to them,
    and not necessarily tell them.
And help me sit, quietly,
    without telling,
    without even squirming to share what I believe
    would be good.

Help me, in my silent support,
    help them allow their answers to come to them.

Let it come to me.

Help me honor—even if I don't understand—
  the process of focusing on this moment's effort
  and trusting God's Universe to fill my heart and hands
  and being
  with abundance.

Help me appreciate and trust—even if I don't understand—
  the synergy of my efforts
  and my belief, my faith,
  with the abundance of the universe.

Help me suspend disbelief
  so that I may make room for all that awaits me
  even as I remain unmoving in my work.

Help me embrace—even if I don't understand—
  the seeming inconsistency
  of being unmoving in action.

Help me act as if I get it
  and keep putting one foot in front of the other,
  doing what I need to do to get where I need to be,
  without letting my goal get in the way of doing what I
    need to do.

DOES THAT MAKE ANY SENSE AT ALL?

It's on the periphery of my understanding.
I'm almost there.
I glimpse getting it.
And then it eludes me.
But with your help,

I will persist
    in my belief,
    in my action,
    in my waiting.

With your help,
    I will let it come to me.

Amen.
Blessings.

Let Them Live!

What songs have inspired you in your life?
For a moment? For a day? for a paper or an essay or an
    article?

What songs do you find yourself singing
    and then realize how they fit your life at this moment?

If not literally or in its entirety, then a word or phrase
    that keeps hitting buttons in you?

Les Mis is one of my favorite musicals—
    overdone, overwrought, over the top of everything,
    but nonetheless, one of my favorites.

It is, first and foremost, based on one of my favorite books—
    Les Miserables which I read in French when I lived in
    Paris.

Even if it were the most terrible of books
    (which it is not),
    it would still rank among my favorites just because of
        the circumstances.

But I digress.

LET THEM LIVE!

Of course, the musical uses the literal meaning of the phrase,
    "Let him live."

It inspired me to go beyond.

How often do I—out of fear, anxiety, wanting to make
    things perfect—
    seek to control the lives and choices of my sons?

I believe (I hope.) that I've evolved to the point
    where I'm AWARE that I want to do this,
    but don't really want to because their lives are theirs,
    and so I pause to breathe deeply
    and move along or away as the situation requires.
Let them live.

Blessed Mother, Holy Spirit,
Lord Jesus,
    All the Angels and Saints and Holy Men, Women, and
        Children,
Help me let them live.
Help me give my best to them as frequently as possible.
Help me lead by GOOD example as best I can.

Help me model the values I seek to instill in them
    because we all KNOW that children model what they
        see and hear;
    they don't follow our instructions
    any more than they come with instructions!

"Do as I say; not as I do" were words I heard frequently
     from my Dad.
This holds a fair amount of wisdom in itself;
     shows awareness of his imperfections
     and idiosyncrasies that he did not want us to repeat.

So, help me. Guide me.
I need to know as they grow
     when to step in to directly steer conversations and
                    activities
     and when to observe and discuss later
     and when to simply observe
     because it's THEIR LIVES,
     and not mine.

Help me applaud with no strings attached.
Help me see without judging or making recommendations.
Help me ASK first, "Would you like my input?"
     and help me shut up when their answer is no.

Let them live.

What they are passionate about is none of my affair.
And certainly, what profession they seek is not meant to be
     of MY choosing.

When they were young,
     I had input into their friends.
Now I must trust that this input remains in
     their hearts as they choose their friends today.

When they were little boys,
    I hope that I showed them frequently enough
    the values of kindness, compassion, love, and
           discernment,
    and that it's good to trust and honor yourself.
Because now,
    I must watch and listen.

And yes, pray in confidence
    that the paths they choose
    are healthy;
    that the ways they choose
    reflect their highest, truest selves.

Help me let go of the need to control.
Help me let them live.

Amen.
Blessings.

Letting Go Of The End Result.

We set goals and we set intentions.
We know where we want to go…
We're anxious to get there…
    sometimes SO anxious
    that we get stuck in THEN
    and we neglect NOW.

Blessed Mother, Holy Spirit,
Lord Jesus,
All the Angels and Saints, Holy Men, Women, and Children,

Help me let go of the end result.

Help me focus on what I'm doing right NOW
    and have faith that
    doing great work NOW,
    treating people well NOW,
    taking steps NOW,
    one after another after another
    will take me
    there.

Or let me see
    that the path of doing NOW
    may take me someplace even better
    than I'd originally intended.

Guide me in my quest to get there
    by focusing on what I'm doing now
    and on being with the people
    I'm with now.

Amen.
Blessings.

LOST!

A day like any other day
    could be
    that the sun is shining inside
    and raining out;

Or

    it could be that the sun is shining outside
    and the rain is pouring down
    on my head and in my heart.

When the center
    is joy,
    I can claw my way out.

I. need. to. get. to. that. center.

It takes…awareness.
It takes…a friend.
It takes…gratitude.
It takes…commitment.
It takes…prayer.

It happens…
    that I feel overwhelmed
    and/or tired
    and/or lonely

and/or less than
and/or behind in my work
and/or unfocused
and/or like the mom in transition that I am
and/or frustrated by what I canNOT do
and/or LOST.

Blessed Mother, Holy Spirit,
Lord Jesus,
    All the Angels and Saints and Holy Men, Women, and
        Children,

Help me be aware.

Guide me to recognizing the signs
    and hear the thoughts
    and the words as they tumble from my lips..
    help me identify the habits of thinking,
    speaking, reacting,
    the old smothering the newer.

Show me the physical signals
    that reflect
    my inner turmoil building.

Show me…so that I may see
    and take care of me
    BEFORE
    I stumble again over my heart
    and end up on the path of belittlement,
    the way of ritualistic self-criticism and judgement,
    the road to self-destruction.

Feed the piece of my mind and heart
     that relies on you for its courage and commitment.
Lead me by the hand
     to rest, to sleep, to self-care
     so that I may shore myself up against
     the habits that so undermine my days and my dreams.

Push me forward to listen to music that buoys the spirit,
     to read the books that soothe the soul and the mind.

Lift my wrist to make a call
     or text or message
     to a friend who will hold a mirror
     before my clouded vision
     and remind me of who I am,
     and what I've done
     and what I will do.

Massage my jaw
     until the words spill out
     and I ask that friend for what I want—
     an umbrella
     to shelter me from the rain of terror
     that I'm tempted to unleash upon my self
     and that I'm working so hard to subdue.

Open my palms
     to receive what my friend offers me.

Open my mind
     to receive your directions.

Open my heart
     to receive the expansion
     that your grace brings.

Amen.
Blessings.

Make My Own Weather.

If you've been following the weather in the midwestern part
    of the United States, you know that winter is just not
        ready
    to let go of us this year.

Snow on May 15?

It happens. It happened yesterday.

This morning, the sun is brilliant.
The birds are singing what I believe is their spring song.
The grass is emerald green.

And it's scheduled to stay cold.

So what? I ask.
I make my own weather.
I carry the sun inside of me
    to share with all whose paths I cross.

Blessed Mother, Holy Spirit,
Lord Jesus,
    All the Angels and Saints and Holy Men, Women, and
        Children,

Guide me as I feed that sunshine.
Help me share the sun and the warmth
wherever I go.

Help me spread the sunshine
with a smile that's based in love and warmth.

No matter the storm around me,
let me shine that sun from within.

Allow me to live Mother Teresa's words
so that everyone may feel better for having met me.

Help me keep that calm, soft, warm demeanor
of the sunny morning
and carry it throughout my day.

Help me make my own weather
and let the storms and cold go wherever they want.

For I have summer's ease and softness and sun
within.

Amen.
Blessings.

Making Rituals From Routines

Making routines and chores into rituals
    clears a space in my mind and heart
    for these rituals to shape and form me
    as well as I them.

I was lead to this place
    of appreciating every day moments,
    including and especially chores
    by genetics, yoga, meditation, Buddhist principles,
    by spiritual practice,
    and by my friend Jacqui,
    whose Intentional Nexting practices
    are magical.

I see and feel and KNOW their value.
I get it.

But oh my goodness how challenging it can be
    when, at each corner,
    lies in wait
    a monster from my past,
    my present,
    but NOT to be of my future.

Blessed Mother, Holy Spirit, Lord Jesus, All the Angels and
    Saints,
    Holy Men, Women, and Children,

Cleaning is therapy.
Cleaning is cleansing.
Cleansing is liberating.
Reframing routine to ritual is glorious.

As I wash my floors today,
    a "task" that taunts and haunts me
    and from which I avert my gaze,
    open my eyes to see
    that washing my floor
    with the clear intention
    of sweeping and washing away
    the old and negative ideas that get in the way
    of me being all I am,
    achieving all I desire.
I open my whole being to the sovereignty
    with which I owe myself and my world
    to live.

The intentional cleansing,
    the ritual of washing
    clears a way through my vulnerability
    to those thoughts and habits of joy and delight
    that allow me to stand in the sparkle
    of my desires and dreams,
    to meet and embrace them as they come to me

    without impairment of detritus of any kind.

This intention
    made each time
    with perhaps the same or different focus

wraps me in its warmth,
opens my eyes, my heart, my whole self.

I thank you for being kindly present
   with me
   as I live each moment with intention,
   as I create the space around me
   to welcome
   all that is.
   and all that I see as my next me.

Amen.
Blessings.

Paralyzed.

What happens
    when
    life spills over the edge of your cup
    and beyond
    where you feel you can flow?

What do you do
    when
    the events of the moment
    pile on top
    of the events of the lifetime
    and you?

What?

"Run away!"
    jumps to mind.

"Shut up!" or shutdown
    are, I suppose,
    other forms of "run away."

Blessed Mother, Holy Spirit,
Lord Jesus,
    All the Angels and Saints and Holy Men, Women, and
        Children,

Hold my hand, please,
    as I navigate these terrifyingly turbulent waters.

Hold my heart, please
    as I weave in and out of
    my mind's traffic
    to find that space of quiet
    that I reserve for moments like this
    but seems just around the corner
    no matter where I turn
    right now.

Hold my soul,
    please,
    as I work desperately
    to honor…
    first, to FIND,
    then to honor
    answers that will best fit
    my truest self.

Tumult rages.
Collapsing in tears
    holds promise…
    momentarily…
    but, of course,
    brings only pounding headaches
    and not relief
    from the image

    that is making me turn
    my gaze away.

I must look.
I must see.
I must step into the hole
    to know and understand.
    I must have you at my shoulder
    to cheer me on
    as I cheer others.

I must tap deeper reserves
    than I'm aware I have
    and for that,
    I rely on you.

My reserves lie beyond me,
    to the shore
    where you stand
    and from which all can be trusted
    to bring peace
    when I look for peace
    in whatever is happening in this moment.

Thoughts swell
    and waves of emotion
    begin to sweep me away.

And I stand strong and tall,
    stubbornly calling on Thich Nhat Han's words:

"I am a mountain—
    strong, tall, imperturbable,
    rigorous, alive;
    the waves of emotion
    can never carry me away."

Steadfast.
Centered.
Doing the dance of old and new,
      then and now.

I reach away from the myth of the sun;
I stretch out to fly higher
than I think I can.
I think I can.

Please help
      me see
      beyond.

Amen.
Blessings.

Prayer For The New Year.

Blessed Mother, Holy Spirit,
Lord Jesus,
> All the Angels and Saints and Holy Men, Women, and
> Children,

Guide me as I step into this New Year.

Help me start each thought, each word, each action
> from a place of love.

Help me believe all that I need to believe
> in order to move with my unique purpose and grace
> to where I must be.

Help me love.
Help me see and receive love when it comes to me.

Help me be open to all the abundance that God spreads
> before me
> and help me accept God's gift.

Help me see my path
> and step into it.

Help me let go of what does not serve my purpose.

Help me know my purpose,
    believe in my purpose,
    pursue my purpose
    with laser-like determination and focus,
    independent of any outside approval
    or fear of disapproval.

Help me identify my fears
    and face them
    with confidence
    that they serve a purpose as well.
Help me learn from them.

Help me learn from all and every.
Help me serve others in the ways
    that THEY need,
        whether or not it's what I would have them need or
            want or be.

Help me be present.
Guide me.
Hold my heart in your gentle hands
    and help me see and free myself
    to be and honor my truest self
    and that of others.

Amen. Amen. Blessings.

Precision.

It's funny.
I've gone through life to date
    (I'm 56.)
    meandering here,
wandering there.
And then I asked myself:
    What DO I want?

And I struggle to answer the questions:

    What is my purpose?
    What do I want
        to be
        to do
        to have.

Choices abound.
I recognize that I can make many things happen.

But what do I WANT?

My mentor and yoga teacher says,
"Ask for what you want."

But what do I WANT?
Blessed Mother, Holy Spirit,
Lord Jesus,

All the Angels and Saints and Holy Men, Women, and
Children,

Help me see into my heart of hearts
shedding expectations,
predictions,
assumptions.

Grant me precision
of vision
of purpose
of desire
of heart
of mind
of spirit.

Help me see
my dreams
so that I may live them exactly as they appear
to me.

Help me
identify
with precision and certainty
what is in my heart
so that
what I create
serves the purpose
I am here to fulfill.

Help me lift
the veils,

the layers,
the ropes that keep me from my vision.

And let me SEE
without the shadows
without the doubt
without the distortion
and with the sweetness
that comes with recognition
of a lifelong friend.

Help me see the forest
AND the trees

That are me.

Amen.
Blessings.

Protect My Mindset.

Where our thoughts go, so do we.
When our thoughts are uplifting,
    we are uplifted and can, therefore,
    be uplifting to those around us.

Precious. It is precious.

Even as I work to express this,
    words stumble over the presence
    in my mind
    of those who judge.
And whose judgment I allow
    to restrain me, keeping me from…me!

Blessed Mother, Holy Spirit,
Lord Jesus,
    All the Angels and Saints and Holy Men, Women, and
        Children,

Help me.
Guide me.
Show me how to stay in beauty,
    stay in peace,
    stay centered in faith,
    in You,
    in me,
    in others.

Help me feel in every cell
     the beliefs that power me to act.
Help me hold in a warm embrace
     the thoughts that empower me
     to do what I believe,
     to do what is right and good and real.

Help me resist those whose shaky faith
     tears into their heart
     and mires them in their misery,
     their hopelessness,
     their inaction.

Help me lead those who are ready, out.
Help me sustain my mindset in the face of those
     who choose—for whatever reason—
     to stay mudbound.

And help me stay strong so that I may persist
     in every goal that holds meaning for me.

No matter how high.
No matter how far away.
No matter how seemingly impossible.

Help me feel the power and rhythm
     of those goals.
Let my faith draw me forward and outward
     and upward.

And beyond.
Beyond my limited and limiting experiences and thoughts.

Help me protect my mindset
    of faith and belief and seeing beauty
    where others see not.

Shore up my defenses
    without building walls that are so impenetrable
    as to isolate me from those whom I would serve.

Help me serve
    without losing a beat of my North star focus.
Help me believe…
    and let that belief carry me beyond where I've
    ever been.

Help me shield my mindset
    from the naysayers,
    and the doubters,
    and the fearful,
    from the darker me.

Help me be fearLESS
    as I step forward and around
    and through
    all the obstacles that I and others
    have put before me through the years.

When I have but a tenuous hold
    on my faith,
    send in reinforcements.

Help me ask others who I know share the struggle,
 and still others who have gone beyond the struggle
 and stand tall and proud and centered in their
 belief.
Protect my mindset
 in ways, please, that allow me to
 celebrate and protect others' mind sets as well.

Let that mindset
 remind me all days
 to intentionally place a smile
 behind my eyes,
 behind my lips,
 behind my heart.

And let those smiles wash over and through me
 to keep me in my faith,
 to help me shine my light,
 to help me keep moving in the direction of…

Amen.
Blessings.

Remember My Why.

How many times
    have I walked up the stairs only to forget
    why I did that?

How many times have I started one project,
    gotten distracted and
    begun working on something else?

How many times?

Countless.

Why am I doing what I'm doing?

It seems to me
    in my more focused moments
    that when I'm able to remember WHY I'm doing
    what I'm doing
    I'm better able to keep going;
    I'm better able to be consistent and persistent.

But, oh!
    keeping my feet firmly planted in the batter's box
    is soooo challenging!

Blessed Mother, Holy Spirit,
Lord Jesus,
All the Angels and Saints and Holy Men, Women, and
Children,

Please help me remember my why;
please help me turn my attention back—
again and again, as many times as it takes—
to my reasons for choosing what I'm choosing.

Steer my thoughts back to my boys
and what I intend to do for them;
back to my husband
and what I intend to do for him;
back to my life
and what I intend to create….
and why!

When the shiny new ideas and toys
come bounding into my field of vision,
help me glance at them,
ask how they could serve my why
and then either integrate them into my plan
or discard them.

Help me do this again and again
because again and again,
I'm faced with some new book to read,
some new program to learn,
some new project to undertake,
some new something
that distracts me from my real why.

Help me remember that
    I can do lot, but I can't do everything
    and do it all or any of it all.

Help me discipline myself to ask:
How does it serve my why?
And if does, ask what it can replace.
And if it does not, let it go.
And let go of the regret that accompanies
    the letting go.

One of my absolute favorite parts of the movie,
    Field of Dreams,
        is when Dr. Graham knows that if he steps over the foul
            line,
        he can never go back to that field of dreams,
        but a child needs his care
        and so, he steps over the line to help her.
With no regrets.
Because he knew his purpose and his why.

And he was at peace with both.

Help me let my why be my north star,
    and my life the compass that perennially
    turns toward that star.

And help me be at peace with my why.

Amen.
Blessings.

Resist the Resistance.

I've been reading this book—

The War of Art: Break Through the Blocks and Win Your Inner Creative Battles

—by Stephen Pressman.

Here's one passage from his book:

"The most pernicious aspect of procrastination is that it can become a habit.
We don't just put off our lives today;
we put them off til our death bed.

Never forget: This very moment, we can change our lives.

There never was a moment, and never will be, when we are

without the power to alter our destiny. This second,

we can turn the tables on Resistance."

These are powerful words.
They remind us of the power within us.

Blessed Mother, Holy Spirit,
Lord Jesus,
    All the Angels and Saints and Holy Men, Women, and
        Children,
Oh…..pleeeeease help
    me resist the resistance.

Help me identify its sources
    and when I can't identify its source immediately,
    let me withstand it
    and DO what it is I intend to do.

Help me succeed
    in ignoring the attraction of this monstrous
    roadblock:

When I start cleaning closets,
    or cleaning…period,
    help me recognize that resistance
    has kicked in and is keeping me from
    my goals.

Help me struggle successfully
    to combat the beast that beckons
    to chocolate or tv or even a book,
    when it is not what I intended to do.
Nudge me, shove me, playfully slap my hand…
    do what it takes to help me resist the resistance

    so that I can create fully,
    wholly, energetically, with laser focus
    and one step at a time,
    with patience and diligence,

with commitment and persistence
and consistency.
Those are the weapons
that I ask you to help me cultivate
as I withstand,
as I resist the resistance
within.

Amen.
Blessings.

Say I.

For years,
    whenever I spoke to groups—
    small or big—
    I spoke in general terms:
    "you," "we," "one"
    (though I may be the only person who still uses that
        expression).

To really face one's demons as well as one's gifts
    (See what I mean?)
    one needs to own them.

I need to say I, me, mine.

When I speak of the need for patience,
    and I use the words "you" or "we,"
    I'm hiding.
When I use the words, "you" or "we,"
    I'm not ready to be naked in my need
    or shame or my despair…
    or my joy!
I'm still timidly tiptoeing around my emotions.

Perhaps it's age,
    perhaps it's experience,
    perhaps the stars are all in the right place—
    I recognize that I've been parading

just as the Emperor in his new clothes,
my faults and failings and gifts and talents
evident
and still I kept trying to hide behind
the ubiquitous YOU.

There is no "I" in TEAM. It's true.
But if the individuals on the team do not know,
    honor, respect, and live their responsibility,
    there is no success in that team either.

When we teach children in developmentally appropriate
    settings
    (My sons are blessed to be with such teachers;
    our schools are not necessarily those places.),
    we start teaching them with the first person—who am
        I?—
    and then stretch out to explore the world
    in ever-expanding circles—
    family, friends, neighborhood, community, city, state,
        country, world.
The buck stops here.
So, I ask for help because it's not easy
    to look in the mirror
    with a loving eye
    and see the stark, raw, honest version
    of yourself...oops...myself
    and not hide in the closet for fear of being frightfully
        ugly.

Blessed Mother, Holy Spirit,
Lord Jesus,
    All the Angels and Saints and Holy Men, Women, and
        Children,

Help me stand up
    and own my feelings—
    fear, mirth, longing, happiness, joy, impatience,
    love, patience, determination, passion, weariness,
    exasperation, tenderness—

Help me own ALL of them
    with equanimity.

Help me hold my gaze
    and not look away in embarrassment or shame.

For there is no shame
    in feeling as I feel.
When I acknowledge and accept,
    I become capable of doing…
    perhaps the same way,
    perhaps differently.

With Your Guidance,
    I step into my self and own
    all that I am—the good, the bad, the ugly, the
        indifferent,
    the beautiful.

With Your Support,
    I use myself as the shining example
    so that others feel
    empowered,
    emboldened,
    encouraged to say, "I."

With Your Love,
    I honor myself and others
    by saying,

"I."

Amen.
Blessings.

See My True Image in the Mirror.

One of the hardest things in life,
    I have found,
    is to look,
    REALLY look,
    in the mirror,
    into my heart of hearts
    and see and hear
    what I have done…

    especially when what I have done
    has undermined my mission,
    my purpose,
    my raison d'être…

    and I don't want to see,
    refuse to see.

No matter what my intention was,
    I need to ask myself,
"What was the end result?"

The best intentions can lead me
    into places
    that appear shiny and new and beautiful and glorious…
    and the shininess dims considerably
    when I look and see the shorn locks
    all over the floor.

One of the hardest things
    is to look myself in the eyes
    and deep into the soul
    and allow myself to see
    that those I call haters—
    because they called out to me
    to bring my attention to what I was really doing
    and not what I imagined or pretended to be doing—
    those "haters" are really the ones
    who persisted in loving me...
    enough to stop what they were doing
    and out to me
    to tell me what they saw.

They stepped out of the dance
    and touched my shoulder
    to speak lovingly to me
    to tell me.

And I deny them
    because I don't want to know.

I call them names
    because I don't want to see.

I lock my arms with the champions
    of my newfound popularity/wealth/knowledge

    because I don't want to acknowledge
    my human-ness.

I turn my head away from the image in the mirror
    that is less than perfect.

I don't want to own my shortcomings,
    faults, failings...

I don't want to face the song of my soul
    because the music I'm dancing frenetically to
    is pulsing and dramatic and vibrant.

Ah...but I DO.

So...
Blessed Mother, Holy Spirit,
Lord Jesus,
    All the Angels and Saints and Holy Men, Women, and
        Children,

I beg of you:
Help me look hard into the eyes staring back at me,
    defying me.

Help me step from behind my words decrying the haters
    into the light of recognizing when I have fallen
    away from my purpose.

Help me stand—
    alone, perhaps,
    in shame, probably,
    in embarrassment, likely.

But help me stand.
Help me soften my heart
    and hear the words
    of those who are brave enough to speak
    the holy words of truth.

Help me open my eyes and ears
    to see and hear the songs
    of those courageous enough to
    take the chance of losing my affection

    so that I may find my path again.

Help me see my true image in the mirror—
    the whole view,
    the entire picture
    so that I may see the shadows behind my eyes
    and heart
    and correct my direction.

Help me put on whatever lenses I need
    to see without the distortions
    of my ego.

Help me look at my truest self,
    my truest purpose,
    my truest mission,
    and hear, really hear,
    and see, really see
    what I'm doing.

Help me draw from that reflection
    looking back at me
    the woman behind the mask,
    the woman beyond the ego,
    the woman who abides in my heart of hearts
    and sometimes needs those "haters"
    to step up and shake my shoulders
    to draw me back into my real self.

Help me see, really see, lovingly see
    my true image in the mirror.

Amen.
Blessings.

Shedding Shame

Upside down
    I am.

Thoughts cartwheeling and spinning
    first to this
    then to that
    then to all at the same time, it feels.

And then nowhere.

Centering
    seems IMPOSSIBLE…
    as my mind
    and heart
    careen from one side of my mind
    to the other and back again.

I can't even keep track of what the thoughts
    are/were
    or
    where I was headed while I was thinking them.

The spinning is making me nauseous.
With anxiety.
With shame. (What is THIS about?!)
With more anxiety about where it's all coming from
    and where it will all go…

Blessed Mother,
    Holy Spirit,
    Lord Jesus,
    All the Angels and Saints
    and Holy Men, Women, and Children,

WHERE ARE YOU?

I'm here.
I think.

Too much, I think.

Help me please sort this out.
Or at least help me stop the spinning
    so that I may sit and breathe.

No.
Help me breathe so that I may stop the spinning
    and sort this out.

Or not.

But DO help me breathe
    slowly
    long
    evenly
    deeply.

Jumbled
    I feel tumbled around
    from here to there and nowhere.

So would you place your hand on my heart
	and sing sweetly
	songs of peace
	and calm
	and remembering?

Life events.
Life changes.
Life losses.
Life gains.

Life…

It IS ever-changing.
And if you would help me relocate my anchor
	in my heart of hearts,
I would SO appreciate it.

If you would help me stand still,
	unwavering in the waves of change,
	yet free to flow with these same waves
	to go where they lead
	and come to terms with where I seek to go?

THIS would be a great gift
	to share.

I'm here.
I know you are too.
My eyes are veiled
	with sweet and sour and wondering and joyful and
		grateful tears.

Help me let them be.
Help me see beyond and around and through them
    to the light,
    to the brilliantly shining light
    of this moment,
    shedding fear,
    shedding sadness,
    shedding anxiety,
    shedding expectation,
    shedding shame,
    shedding disappointment,
    shedding.

Just shedding.

Amen.
Blessings.

Smile!

Research shows us that the body believes
    everything we say, think, hear.

Research also tells us that
    we alter our brain chemistry by changing our
        thoughts…
    and by changing our body.

For example,
    people who were told to frown
    did so,
    and then experienced a downshift in their mood;
    told to smile,
    they did that and experienced upshift in their mood.

So, by putting a smile on my face,
    I raise my energy level,
    I elevate my mood;
    I feel better, more positive, more in control.

Blessed Mother, Holy Spirit,
    Lord Jesus,
    All the Angels and Saints and Holy Men, Women, and
        Children,

Help me put a smile on my face.

Help me recognize
    that I control my mood,
    my approach to life,
    my responses to people around me—
    no matter what.

Help me set the intention every day
    to put a smile behind my eyes,
    behind my lips, behind my heart.

Help me appreciate
    the impact that my smile
    has on me
    AND the world around me.

Help me take the initiative
    to smile
    and to trust the power
    of my mind/body/spirit
    to change my world
    and thus,
    change the world around me.

Abraham Lincoln wrote:
    "Folks are as happy as they make up their minds to be."

Help me force that smile
    when I'm feeling blue,
    and have faith
    that my mouth smiling
    will help the rest of me
    feel better.

Really.

Smile and the world smiles with you.

Amen.
Blessings.

Soften My Heart.

Antoine de Saint-Exupery
wrote in The Little Prince,

"It is only with the heart that one can see rightly;
what is essential is invisible to the eye."

Pema Chodron
reminds us not to let
"life harden our heart."

It's easier, of course,
to say then do.
I have lots of reasons—we all do—
for putting armor around my heart.
I've experienced lots of hurts and disappointments,
betrayals, denials, fears.

Nonetheless,
the only purpose the armor serves
is to perpetuate more of the same.

It sure seems like it protects us from the arrow
and barbs and sticks and stones.

In reality,
our hurt, our broken-heartedness

links us to all the others in the world
who have ever loved.
And when we embrace it, sit with it,
    our broken heart teaches us to love.

In reality,
    our soft heart,
    the chinks in the armor,
    open us to compassion.

And so I ask,
    Blessed Mother, Holy Spirit,
    Lord Jesus,
    All the Angels and Saints and Holy Men, Women, and
        Children,

Help me soften my heart
    and release the armor around it.

Help me sit
    with my hurt and disappointment
    rather than banish it
    and transmute it to hardness, bitterness,
    resentment or blame.

Help me feel the pain
    and learn its lessons of forgiveness.

Help me see
    that a soft heart, its vulnerability,
    make me strong
    rather than weak.

Help me know
   that compassion holds more promise
   than judging, criticizing,
   shaming others or myself.

Help me act on that soft and open heart.
Help me hold out its promise to others
   instead of turning my head to their distress
   or lecturing them on their errors.

Help me acknowledge and accept
   that this soft heart is my true nature
   and the true nature of others as well;
   that to live from and celebrate
   and cultivate my soft heart
   is to live my truest self.

Help me follow the steps of
   Mother Teresa,
   for example,
   who understood,
   and devoted her life to demonstrating this truth.
Help me uncover in my own heart
   this spot of tenderness
   and help me practice compassion, loving-kindness, joy
   and equanimity
   that gives me greater access to that spot.

Help me soften…soften…soften…
   help me love.

Amen.
Blessings.

Sparkle.

One of the gifts of a frigidly cold winter
    is that, on days when the sun is shining,
    I can see the air sparkle,
    alight with the sun and the cold.

I can see the light glimmer
    on the frozen branches
    and twinkle
    in the icicles dangling
    from the eaves.

It reminds me to animate my life
    with brilliance.

Blessed Mother, Holy Spirit,
    Lord Jesus,
    All the Angels and Saints and Holy Men, Women, and
        Children,

Nudge me to look and to see
    the beauty around me.

Help me see past my discomfort in the cold
    to experience the breathlessness
    of watching the air flash and flicker
    with the sunlight all around me.

Remind me
    to pause and allow myself to be dazzled
    by this sparkle.

Remind me
    to pause
    and see the shimmer in my own spirit
    and the radiance in my own self.

Help me to identify with all the beauty
    around me
    so that I may see and feel
    the beauty within me.

Draw me into the sparkle
    so that I feel part of its brilliance,
    your brilliance
    and my own.

Amen.
Blessings.

Speak My Truth With Gentleness.

"We all have truths; are mine the same as yours?"
Herod sings these words in the rock opera *Jesus Christ
Superstar*.

They echo across our lives as our paths cross with folks
from different families, different neighborhoods,
different worlds.

We all deserve to speak our truth.

If we truly believed in our heart of hearts
that we deserve to speak our truth,
we wouldn't need to express that truth
with the anger, hostility, and meanness
that we tend to use.

We defy people to listen to us.

And in doing so, we undermine our desire to speak our
truth
and to be *listened to* as we speak.

Who wants to listen to anything that
is spoken with hostility, anger, meanness

Blessed Mother, Holy Spirit,
     Lord Jesus,
     All the Angels and Saints and Holy Men, Women, and
          Children,

Help me first, believe that I deserve to know and speak my
     truth.

And failing that, help me fake it til I make it:

Help me speak my truth
     with gentleness and grace,
     with kindness and with an open heart
     so that my words, my truth,
     can sneak out from behind my armor
     and penetrate the armor of those
     to whom I'm sharing my truth.

Turn my eyes away from my fears of not being heard
     or respected or honored
     and help me honor and respect myself
     so that I may speak
     with faith in myself,
     in my truth.

Change my gaze so that it begins inward
     and then carries my words with
     unwavering confidence
     to the ears and hearts of those I wish to tell my truth to
     and those who wish to listen.

Help me fill my gaze with intention
    of speaking clearly,
    even lovingly
    as my voice communicates
    the passion behind my words
    and not the fear of being dismissed
    or berated.

Help me place into my voice
    my conviction
    without hostility;
    my passion
    without fear;
    my truth
    without daring those around me to
    defy me.

Help me place my truth on the table,
    calmly
    and without wanting anything in return.
Help my hands and voice reflect the honor
    and respect that I give myself
    and those whose attention I desire.

Those who listen
    will respond to my manner
    before they hear my words.

Help me do everything I can
    to make my manner consistent with my words
    and my words consistent with my truth.

Help me speak my truth
　　with greater gentleness and grace.

Amen.
Blessings.

The I in Team.

We're told—repeatedly—
   that there is no "I" in "team."

Clearly, the successful team
   is one where everyone works towards the same goal,
   with no egos to clutter their path
   to winning.

I believe that the successful team
   is one where
   each teammates knows the value of "I."

And knows and accepts his/her responsibility
   totally and completely.

I believe that a successful team
   is where all of the "I"s step up and into their game,
   bringing their finest gifts, finest work,
   finest effort
   to the team.

The successful team is composed of "I"s
   and not egos.

The successful team
   knows how to work together;

the stars help everyone to be stars,
the leaders DO rather than tell.

In a word,
    members of the successful team
    say I.

Blessed Mother, Holy Spirit,
    Lord Jesus,
    All the Angels and Saints and Holy Men, Women, and
        children,

Help me step up and say, "I."

Help me see, acknowledge, accept, celebrate
    what I bring to the game—
    strengths and weaknesses—
    so that I really am an asset
    to my teams.

Help me see
    that my teams—
    family, staff, friends,
    students, clients, colleagues, community—
    need me to be real,
    to be honest,
    to be true.
Help me see that.
Help me do that.
Help me see that when I say, "I,"
    I open myself to all possibilities
    of abundance.

Help me see that when I say, "I,"
　　the world releases blessings
　　and prosperity beyond imagination
　　beyond what I might achieve alone.

Help me see that when I say, "I,"
　　my team soars
　　high above the average score;
　　and help me see that
　　it is in helping the other "I"s on my team,
　　that I reach my truest potential.

Help me see that
　　to succeed on a team
　　and with a team,
　　there must be an "I"
　　before there can be a "we."

And help me see and help others see
　　that this I
　　is the truest, highest self
　　that steps up and answers,
　　and says,
　　"I."
So that
　　we may say we.

Amen.
Blessings.

The Song In My Heart.

Each day these days
    I get up and thank God for all that I am,
    all that I have, all that I learn.

An attitude of gratitude, after all,
    catapults us to greater heights and depths of spirit
    than we reach without an awareness of and appreciation
        for
    the gifts we are given
    even when those gifts are wrapped in ugly paper.

And then, I ask,
What is my purpose?
What is my intention?
What is my mission?
What is the song in my heart?
    of my heart?

Do you know the song in your heart?
Can you sing along?
Does the music make your heart soar
    and your spirit smile wide
    with openness and love?
    resolve and determination?

Blessed Mother, Holy Spirit,
  Lord Jesus,
  All the Angels and Saints and Holy Men, Women, and
    Children,

Help me hear the music, my music,
  feel its tempo and rhythm.
Help me tap my toes to its beat.
Help me get up and dance when the melody
  moves me to do so.

Help me listen also with full attention
  to all the silent moments of that song
  —not to fill those moments,
  but to leave them empty
  in order to create the space for the music to exist,
  to flourish,
  to exalt in the compositions that flow from within.

Help me see myself as the virtuoso
  of my life, the composer, the producer, director,
    musician,
  audience…all in one
  and appreciate whatever sounds come forth.
Let those sounds
  and whatever form they take—
  jazz, fusion, classical, blues, R & B,
  rock, chamber, country, bluegrass,
  big band, hip-hop, rap—
  lead me to their Source.

Let me understand that the music in me
  is me.

And let me embrace the song in my heart,
    the music of my soul,

    as well as the song in your heart
    so that we might harmonize our joyful noise.

Amen.
Blessings.

The Truth About Me.

One of my greatest challenges in life
    is to learn to look in the mirror
    and see clearly—
    without judging, criticizing, cringing, shaming, or
        blaming—
    what is really there.

To look at my thoughts, words, behaviors,
    tones of voice, postures, prejudices,
    successes, failures, strengths, and weaknesses—
    without defending,
    without accusing—

    is to allow myself to learn from each of them.

When I do that,
    I unburden myself of the lifelong curse
    of perfection.

I allow myself to learn from everything and everyone;
    I allow myself to learn from
    the truth about me.

Blessed Mother, Holy Spirit,
    Lord Jesus,
    All the Angels and Saints and Holy Men, Women, and
        Children,

Hold my hand as I face this strongest of demons—
    the tenacity with which
    I hold onto the myths about myself.

Help me let go of what I grew up with—
    through words that were spoken to me
    or around me,
    through ways that I heard the words
    and viewed the world.

When the night of me seems too dark,
    let me rest against you
    until the light of me awakens
    my awareness of the gifts that are me—
    the truth of me.

Forgive me,
    or better yet,
    help me forgive myself for being human.
Better yet,
    help me see that being human
    is a gift

    so that I may learn from each of the things I do
        and from all of those I do not.

Hiding things away
    gives them such monstrous enormity and power.
The shadows control us
    when we turn from them.

Help me gently remove the veils
    that I mistakenly believe
    hide the ugly, the misshapen, the grotesque.
For when those veils are brushed away,
    and I see the whole panorama,
    the whole inner landscape,
    the details of which have eluded me
    for as long as I've hidden behind those veils,
    I see grace.
    I see beauty.
I see truth and peace and love
    in all of me.

The strengths light the way to see
    the things I call weaknesses.
And when I'm aware of these weaknesses,
    I'm able to learn even more greedily
    and speedily how to cede
    space and time and power to others
    who have the gifts that I do not.
They keep me vulnerable and compassionate
    and aware of others.

And for that I am eternally grateful.

The truth?

The truth is that when I'm able to see and celebrate
    myself as I am,
    I get to see and celebrate others
    as they are.

And then, we can do epic things.

As Macrina Wiedekehr says, "Oh! God, let me believe the truth about myself…

no matter how beautiful it is."

Amen.
Blessings.

Turn Down the Noise.

Turn down the noise.
Turn off the noise.

Others' opinions.
Others' ideas.
Others' impressions.
Others' others' others'...

How many times have I deferred
    to others' thoughts
    because I didn't listen to or trust
    my own?

How often has it happened
    that I missed out on a friendship
    with someone
    because I took others' experiences/opinions
    and held myself back?

Too often.
Countless times.

Blessed Mother, Holy Spirit,
    Lord Jesus,
    All the Angels and Saints and Holy Men, Women, and
        Children,

Help me look with my eyes.
Help me listen with my ears.
Help me see and hear from my heart.

Instead of looking at people, places, things
    through others' eyes,
    with others' ideas,
    guide me around and through
    to the person who stands before ME,
    with ME,
    talking to ME.

Because we're each so wonderfully unique,
    our experiences will ALWAYS be unique to each of us.

Good, bad, or indifferent,
    the experience belongs to you, or him, or her…
    or me!

And that's what I want to respond to.

Guide me.
Help me.
Steer me to a clear perspective
    that is unique to me
    so that I may enjoy the friendship that is unique to me,
    the book or movie or play or song that is unique to me,
    so that I may enjoy the life that is unique to me.

Help me to allow myself
    to see and not judge with someone else's standards.

Paula Strupeck Gardner • 179

Help me discern
>   how the puzzle pieces go together
>   in my puzzle,
>   rather than force someone else's pieces
>   into mine.

And help me be open to the changes
>   that happen each day.
What was true yesterday
>   may be less…or more…true today.

Ah…but that's a prayer for another day!

Help me turn down the noise
>   of the others' words ringing in my head
>   so that I may listen to my own lyrics.

Help me turn down the noise
>   of the others' melodies,
>   sometimes scraping and jarring
>   against my own,
>   so that I may, indeed, hear my own song.

Help me turn off the noise…

Amen.
Blessings.

Turn Your Attention To...

Have you been thinking I've been too busy to share my
    prayers
    the last few days?

Actually,
    I've been too busy dealing with my fear
    to give any attention
    to writing my prayers.

I'm traveling.
And I surprised my husband with a visit
    and a vacation.
And left our younger son on his own
    (with the help of family, friends, and neighbors).

I believe our fears
    can teach us a great deal
    when we acknowledge them,
    explore them,
    address them,

    and let them go
    to turn our attention to what we want
    rather than what we fear.

Blessed Mother, Holy Spirit,
  Lord Jesus,
  All the Angels and Saints and Holy Men, Women, and
    Children,

Help me acknowledge my fears,
  help me address them,
  help me let them go and turn my attention
  to what I'm grateful for,
  to the beauty that I want to create,
  to the purpose with which I live,
  to the wisdom of letting go of the need to control.

We don't, my husband and I,
  as a rule, fly together,
  unless we're flying as a family.
And I'm afraid of dying before I finish my job as mom.
So,
  I pray for inspiration to make arrangements—
  just in case something happens to me.

Because sticking my head in the sand
  does not make it go away
  and NOT planning for contingencies
  would be irresponsible and unfair
  to my sons.

And then I pray for help in letting go
  of those fears.
And I pray for help in turning my attention TO
  my purpose,
  my dreams,
  my intentions.

I ask you to hold my hand
    as I relinquish fear's hold on my heart
    and give my full presence and
    turn my attention
    to this moment.

Help me do what I know will keep me planted
    in now—
    help me breathe deeply,
    help me release the fears,
    help me welcome and settle into gratitude,
    help me refocus on the images of where I'm going
    and feel the feelings that I seek to experience—
    courage, self-confidence, calm, joy, excitement, faith;
    help me remember past moments
    when I've triumphed in the face of fee.
Help me apply all of those strategies
    to now.

Help me acknowledge my fears.
Help me address what needs to be done.
Help me let them go and turn my attention
    to sending out into the universe
    all the energy that I want to receive.

Help me do the right thing for my children
    by taking care of "what if"
    AND
    by being an example of
    living life,
    of creating the life I love,

    of wrapping my fears in wonder.

Amen.
Blessings.

Wake To Peace.

Churning stomach?
Crawling skin?
Mind spinning out of control?

Is this how you feel when the alarm goes off
    to get you going in the morning?
    Or
    is this how you feel when you wake up BEFORE
    the alarm?

Behind your eyes, into your throat, your belly…
    your whole being cringing with an anxiety of an
            unknown
    source.

Maybe you ignore it.
But it follows you into your day.

How to shed that nagging, persistent,
    troublesome concern?

Blessed Mother, Holy Spirit,
    Lord Jesus,
    All the Angels and Saints and Holy Men, Women, and
        Children,

Help me be aware of how the anxiety creeps into my
    dreams and shakes me awake.
Help that awareness lead me to a different space.

With that awareness,
Help me create the peace that I seek to wake to.

Help me breathe
    slow, long, even, deep breaths
    to help release the hold on my mind, my body,
    my spirit.

Help me listen to that breath as I breathe
    instead of sinking into the anxious, tight ball
    that's forming in my belly and my throat.

Help me allow myself to free myself
    from the hold
    of that ball
    by listening to the breath,
    by concentrating my attention on the breath going in
    and going out.

Help me see and feel
    the grip release
    and a sense of peace
    entering my mind, body, spirit.

Remind me of Thich Nhat Han's words:
Breathing in, I relax.
Breathing out, I smile.

Help me smile into the day.

Help me create peace
    so that I may wake to peace
    today.
    tomorrow.
    every day.

Peace.

Amen.
Blessings.

What Can I Bring?

We talk a lot about what we feel from the environment,
　　the energy that we pick up from others,
　　what we absorb from others' words and behaviors.

I'm wondering today:
What am I bringing to the conversation?
What energies am I emitting to others?
What am I sending out into the environment?

And so I pray:
　　Blessed Mother, Holy Spirit,
　　Lord Jesus,
　　All the Angels and Saints and Holy Men, Women, and
　　　　Children,

Help me see what I'm sending out there
　　and help me make it great,
　　peaceful,
　　kind and loving.

Help me start from my heart
　　and speak so that others feel this heart
　　filled with compassion.
Help me fill the room
　　with my loving energy,
　　will, and determination

to contribute good and beauty
to this world.

Let me not rely on others for that energy;
        let me, instead,
        exude all that I wish to see in this world.

When I step into a conversation,
        help me speak from an intention of
        centering on others
        and not of drawing attention to myself.

Help me integrate seamlessly
        into the positive energy out there
        or
        help me draw others into
        positive energy from wherever they are.

What can I bring?
To this room?
To this community?
To this world?

Rather than ask,
What can I have or get?
Let me ask,
What can I give?
What can I bring of goodness and light?

Amen.
Blessings.

What Do I NOT Need Help With?

Blessed Mother, Holy Spirit,
    Lord Jesus,
    All the Angels and Saints, and Holy Men, Women, and
        Children,

Oh.

I sat to meditate today
    and asked the question:
What do I need help with today?

And without a nanosecond of delay,
    the response came:

What do I NOT need help with?

So.

I ask this:

At the moments
    when life seems to be crashing down
    and the disappointments of a lifetime
    knock me about my head and heart;
    when the light
    is completely obscured
    by fears, sorrows, disappointments,

by fears, confusions, misgivings,
        lies,
        by fears…

if I can't make it right at that moment,
if I'm lost in the space of my mind's wanderings,

help me laugh, please.

Help me laugh at the absurdity of it all,
        at the veils that distort my view,
        at the misshapen image in the mirror,
        at the uncertainty and the growling in my heart and
                head,
        at the mind that never. stops. thinking…

which…hmmm…leads to creating.

Help me laugh at rude and insensitive behaviors..

Ah… at our human-ness,
        yours, mine, theirs;

        at my shallow breath
        which I can deepen with awareness…

Yes.

Help me laugh at life.
With life.
With myself.

And that laugh out loud
    has already sparked me to clear my head,
    lighten my heart,
    sweep my sight and vision clean;
    has helped me remember to place a smile
    behind my eyes,
    behind my lips,
    behind my heart…

And feel the softness that moves into
    my thoughts,
    my words,
    my actions.

Ahhhhhh…..men
Blessings.

When Melancholy Visits.

It happens.
Who knows when we'll wake up
    with a sense of sadness, disconnectedness or
    other vague hopelessness gnawing at our consciousness,
    pawing at our mindset,
    insistent in its gloom?

Sometimes, we can identify quickly
    the source of our melancholy —
    a child gone back to school for another semester,
    a disappointment at work,
    loss of a friend,
    illness,
    normal life passage events,
    lack of sleep…

Loss and change and disappointment
    are everywhere in our life
    and part and parcel of who we are as human beings.

Other times, we wonder, we search,
    we explore and find very little in our life
    that leads to this vague sense of sadness
    that is relentless in its ambiguous but wide-reaching
    net of drear.

The blue melody floats through our system,
    insinuating itself into mind and heart,
    while we watch and wonder
    where it came from
    and how to get rid of it.

Sometimes, we fight by pushing it away.
Other times, we deny its existence and its power.
Still other times, we fall into its somber rhythm,
    and we pulse with its mournful dejection
    for days...
    or even months and years.

What do we do to keep melancholy's visit short?
    and reduce its hold on our heart?

Blessed Mother, Holy Spirit,
    Lord Jesus,
    All the Angels and Saints and Holy Men, Women, and
        Children,
Let me see and understand
    the value of embracing the melancholy when it arrives
        on my doorstep
    like a guest who knows it is unwelcome.

Help me sit with melancholy for a bit
    and ask it where it came from,
    what it's about,
    and allow it to answer
    even with responses that I don't care for
    or would rather not see.

Lead me to visit with this misery
    as though it had something of importance to share with
        me
    because it does…
And help me appreciate that when I ignore or deny this
    unwelcome guest,
I give it more power, more control over my mind, my body,
    my spirit
    and increase the likelihood that its stay
    will extend with my resistance.

Help me maintain my friendly awareness
    that melancholy has something
    to share with me
    that is part of being human
    and that can enhance my appreciation for
    the sun shining on my shoulders.

Please help me allow myself
    the equanimity to move step by step,
    side by side
    with melancholy and then
    choose a different, diverging path
    that takes me to a place of recognition
    and gratitude and love.

Help me let that mournfulness go,
    waving a grateful good-bye,
    recognizing that life will undoubtedly
    direct melancholy to my door again
    because life is gain and loss
    and loss and gain.

And help me see beyond and around melancholy's visit
   and remember where it and I come from,
   letting loss be part of the game,
   recognizing the other parts as well
   and living where I am
   in this moment
   neither turning my back on my guest
   nor choosing to allow a long, drawn-out dispirited
         sojourn,

   letting life's flow
   carry away the sadness
   and letting me tap into my joy,
   the jewel inside my heart of hearts,
   recognizing, acknowledging, and welcoming
   my natural state of being.

Amen.
Blessings.

Worthy.

I stumble over these feelings.
I have resisted them
    (seeing them, naming them)
    for months…

No… for a lifetime.

And today,
    they've jumped onto my table
    and into my lap
    and REFUSE to be put down, away, ignored.

They will NOT be ignored;
    because TODAY, they feel threatened;
    they want to win.

They have insinuated themselves
    stealthily,
    silently,
    craftily
    into every thought,
    every word (spoken and unspoken)
    every choice,
    every feeling,
    every action,
    every reaction,
    every response,

every anticipation,
Every. Every. Every.

When you believe that you don't matter,
    that you're unworthy,
    your thoughts and actions scatter easily.
Because to focus
    means to confront the insistent
    pounding on the door,
    telling you,
"Give it up! You cannot do this;
    should not do this because
    you. are. unworthy."
When you're not ready for the confrontation,
    when you're afraid you'll lose,
    that you'll succumb to the voices that echo
    from childhood—

"We heard you the first time. Be quiet."
    (but we chose to NOT acknowledge you
    because you. do. not matter.)

It's TERRIFYING:

Turning your face to the light
    means turning away from a lifetime
    of feeling unworthy, unheard, unworthy of being heard.

Turning your face to the light
    means turning your heart from the cold wall
    of a core belief that repeats that message
    in an amazing variety of forms
    in an amazing variety of messages

in an amazing and complex variety of habits
and rituals and unconscious living.

It looked like this:

~speech so quiet as to be imperceptible—unhearable;

~dress so dark or so beige as to hide the person wearing
    it—never red, please!

~accomplishments, overlooked or left unclaimed
        because to do so would mean arrogance…
        and you. are. unworthy.

~praises denied, diminished;

~silence when your heart was singing with words that
        could bless others' lives
        because
        you.
        are.
        unworthy.

It's been a journey.
It IS a journey.

Today, I stand firm.

Blessed Mother, Holy Spirit, Lord Jesus,
    All the Angels and Saints and Holy Children, Women,
        and Men,

Help. Me. Focus.
Help. Me. Be Aware.

Help me throw my light,
    my brilliance,
    my shining, truest self
    into the darkest corners
And draw the truth
    from them.

Help me silence
    the voices
    that prompted the little girl
    to feel unnecessary, inconsequential, unworthy.

Close my ears and nose and throat and body
    to the insidious messages
    declaring over and over and over:

> *"Whatever you do, you cannot win favor;*
> *whatever you say, you will not be heard;*
>
> *Don't bother trying. Don't bother dreaming.*
>
> *You'll fail.*
>
> *Because You. Are. Unworthy."*

Please, help me
Draw a curtain of steel
    around the lambs with daggers
    hidden in their hard gaze
    and gravelly voice,

those who seek to suffocate the light,
who seek to strangle the voice,
who want my company in the dark
because they couldn't/wouldn't—through their own
history of others blanketing *their* joy—
step into their light
and shine light unto others
or receive others' light to open their path.

Guide my gaze
to the center of this spacious heart
to view,
unveiled, unclouded,
unshadowed,
the clear pool of love
that resides there,
always has,
always will.

Lead me,
through awareness,
to another place,
not of blame,
nor of shame,
but of light.

As the light expands,
let it warm and comfort,
let it inspire and illuminate the path to my soul,
so that I may see
the dark beliefs that have haunted me

and release them....

to the light.

Because
I. Am. Worthy.

Amen.
Blessings.

Vaccination Against Self-Sabotage.

Oh! how often I have stepped on my toes
    (There's a more colorful expression,
    but I'll save it for conversation!)!

Oh! how frequently I work against myself
    as I work for myself...

So I'm stuck,
    spinning my wheels,
    getting nowhere
    in a push-me/pull-you position,
    mired in that no-mans-land
    of desire and self-doubt;
    ambition and self-sabotage.

Blessed Mother, Holy Spirit,
    Lord Jesus,
    All the Angels and Saints and Holy Men, Women, and
        Children,

Help me out of this destructive rut.
Help me reformat and restructure my brain
    to allow me to step onto the playing field
    with all systems focused on success.

Squeeze my hand to remind me to exercise
    the strength of will
    to refocus
    away from the self-destructive, undermining
    patterns of thought and behavior
    and toward the light of Your truth for me,
    for all of us.

Help me accept that I am worthy;
    that I am lovable;
    that I am capable
    and that my thoughts help or hurt me
    depending on which I allow to linger.

Tap my arm
    to get my attention off of my traditional thoughts of, "I
        can't"
    or "how" or "what makes me think I should."

Help me reroute my attention from the limits of my past
    to the abundance of my future.

Give me that shot of faith
    that has in the past been labelled "Pollyana-ism,"
    but that merits focus
    for all the good thing it brings
    to those who believe.

Help me shed yesterday's fears.
Let me hold nothing back;
    let me dance all the way through.

Stir the creative juices that are writhing
    to be freed from their prison of habit
    and let them inspire in me ways and means
    to step outside of the ruts of negativity
    and make new pathways.

Turn my eyes toward the light
    that I may follow it, walking and running
    with confidence
    instead of crawling under the weight of confusion
    and disbelief.

Help me be immune
    to the forces that would have me abandon
    myself, my dreams, my visions,
    so that I may stand and speak
    my truth
    with tender and kind conviction.

Vaccinate me against the powerful distractions
    of negativity and doubt and fear
    so that I may see, touch, hear, feel,
    be
    all that I am,
    all that I desire,
    all that I see.

Let me start each day
    with inspiration
    rather than fear;
    with focus
    rather than distraction;

with confidence
rather than confusion.

Let me start each day with and in You.

Amen.
Blessings.

Epilogue

With these prayers, I share with you the depths of my fears so that you may honor your own. I give you my words so that you may use them until you find yours or until you decide to make these words your own.

With this body of prayers, I offer you a way in and a way out— a way into yourself and a way out of whatever steps in your way as you move out from behind your heart and into your light.

I welcome your thoughts, your words, your questions and encourage you to stay in touch with me by joining my email list here.
(https://worthyofwingswithpaulagardner.aweb.page/ Wrapping-Your-Fears-In-Wonder)
(You'll also get a free audio version of the prayer poems!)

We are all blessed by being here.

Amen.
Blessings.

Paula

Acknowledgements

Sir Isaac Newton wrote, "If I have seen further, it is by standing on the shoulders of Giants."

I gratefully acknowledge all of the people who have made my life the blessing it is—my Teachers, my Students, my Parents and Sisters and Brothers, their spouses and their children, my awesome nieces and nephews, my cousins and Aunts and Uncles, my friends and teammates and co-workers, and, of course, my husband and my sons.

You are all my Teachers. And I thank you for it.

I thank Jason Legaard for prompting me to get the first edition OUT THERE. I thank Sandie Nielson for spurring me on to do and not wait. I thank fellow students along the way for helping me open the door and step out into the sunshine to play. I thank Renee McCombs, who opened the window to the online community for me. I thank all my on-and offline friends for responding to my prayers with likes and comments and requests that led me to know that I needed to put this book together. Now. I thank Audrey Vela from the bottom of my heart for caring for our business as her own, allowing me greater freedom to do what I love—write, facilitate, share, repeat!

Yoga and meditation and Ayurveda have brought me focus and peace that have allowed me to pray from my heart to yours.

I thank YOU for being here.

About The Author

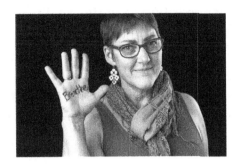

Paula Strupeck Gardner, M.A., M.A. is a Mom In Transition, Still: Her sons have begun their own lives in different cities, the elder one with his beautiful wife.

Paula has been writing since before she knew the words (Her 2-year-old's scribbles are part of the family book collection.) and teaching for almost as long. A former French, ESL, and Linguistics instructor, Paula's favorite teaching experience was that of stay-at-home mom although Paula feels she did more learning than teaching during that time!

Before children, Paula and Jack, her husband of nearly 30 years, travelled extensively, including to run marathons in Nanisivik and Nepal, where Paula was the first-ever US woman to complete the Mt. Everest Marathon in 1989. Although their travelling was different with the boys, they did make time to live with their sons in the south of France for 3 months when the boys were 8 and 10 years old.

Paula now teaches yoga and ayurveda and guides transformational retreats and mini-retreats (in-person and online) for people who enjoy balancing their lives with sound, movement, meditation, and food!

To receive a free recording of Paula reading a prayer poem from this collection and others and Paula's emails about upcoming retreats or to plan one of your own, register at:

https://worthyofwingswithpaulagardner.aweb.page/
Wrapping-Your-Fears-In-Wonder

Paula sees herself as a facilitator of learning and is delighted that so many people have embraced her prayers as reflections of their own hearts and minds.

Friends, family, and students have encouraged her over the years to publish so that everyone could experience the sense of peace that her writing and speaking evokes.

Paula encourages you to listen to your own heart and to the hearts of those around you.

Also by Paula Strupeck Gardner:

MS Chair Yoga At Home Your Step-By-Step Guide 25 Poses To Alleviate Tension, Tightness, & Anxiety So You Can Thrive

Making Sacred Space

My EveryDay Prayer Book Volume II (available in 2021)

My Ministry of Motherhood

Got Back Pain? Get Pain Free!

One Final Prayer

In my chosen work of serving, supporting, and connecting and sharing, I love to receive feedback from my readers and clients and students.

Would you please take a moment to write your honest review of this book?

Go to Amazon and Barnes and Noble and leave your review.

I appreciate your taking the time.

Amen.
Blessings.

Made in the USA
Monee, IL
06 March 2021

62117926R00118